The Metabolic Typing ® Diet Cookbook
for 3-A, Balanced

by Nancy Dale, C.N.

Metabolic Type® and Metabolic Typing® are Registered
Trademarks of Healthexcell

contents

preface   5
foreword   6
acknowledgment   7
introduction   8

glycemic index   10
facts on fiber   12
emotional eating   13
metabolic type   15
foods for your type   18
shopping list   19

begin the day   21
salads and more   33
soups and one pot meals   47
vegetables and more   63
proteins   79
desserts and snacks   103

glossary   115
legend, weight and measures   119
index   121
resources   125

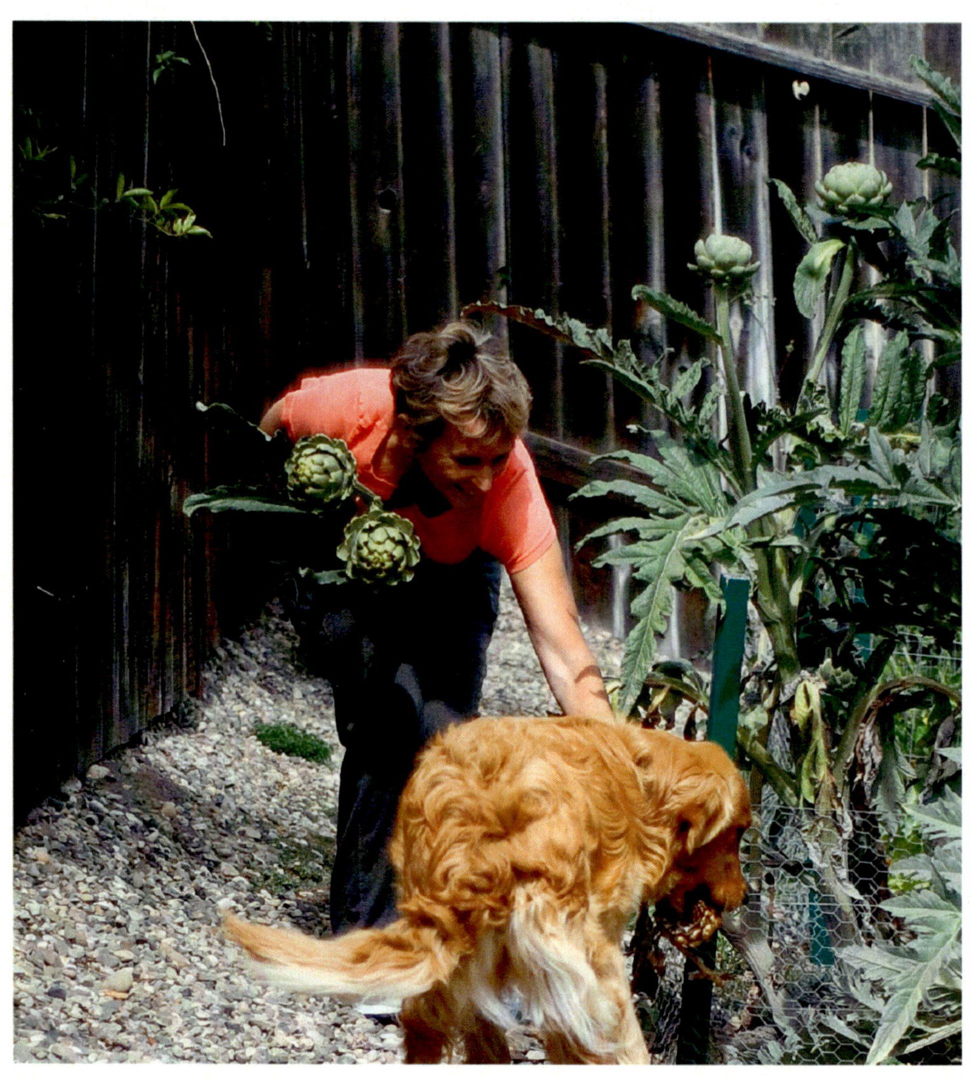

Eating to live, not living to eat.

Preface

This book took over fifteen years to create and I believe it is still a work in progress. I began cooking when I was a small girl. When I became a certified nutritionist I decided to delve into cooking from a health standpoint. Just as I completed my chef certificate in 1994 my mother was diagnosed with liver cancer. I quickly moved in with her and began cooking as a means to bring her back to health. She was given just weeks to live. I lived with her for 5 ½ years cooking all the while.

At that same time I started my clinical nutrition practice. I could only work part time while attending to my mother. I started cooking for my clients to show them what healthy meals taste like and before long I had developed a business of creating healthy meals, delivered to my clients. I lived in the Southern California area and began working with the movie industry. I was hired to work with the stars when their role required them to lose weight or to get healthier. Most of the meals in this book were created at that time.

Since moving to the Santa Barbara area I no longer cook and deliver my food. I now teach cooking classes in my home twice a year and operate two nutrition offices.

 I became a Certified Metabolic Typing ® Advisor five years ago and began creating menus based on that same principle.

All of the recipes in the book have been created with your health in mind. We can not expect restaurants or prepared foods to give us health. It is my hope that you begin to love cooking as much as I do.

Bon appétit!

Nancy Dale, C.N.

Foreword

Over 30 years ago, my sojourn with Metabolic Typing® first began. From the very first encounter, I knew in my heart, in my whole being, that I had been blessed with the good fortune to have found something very special. So intriguing, so rewarding has that 3 decades long journey been, that nothing has been able to entice my one-pointed attention away from my quest to uncover the wondrous and amazing secrets of health possible through Metabolic Typing®.

As might be imagined, a lot can happen over 3 decades – or over half a lifetime in my case. And so it has. Just like the accidental discovery of a piece of a broken pot can lead to an anthropological dig that unearths an entire ancient city, what began as a one dimensional concept to determine individual dietary requirements has evolved, one discovery at a time, into an 11 dimensional model for the science of optimal health known as Metabolic Typing®.

The complexity, depth and breadth of this scientific discipline is staggering, when understood in its entirety. And yet, the day-to-day application of the truths revealed through Metabolic Typing® is utterly simple, once you know exactly what to do and how to do it.

Through the <u>Metabolic Typing® Cookbooks</u>, Nancy Dale has provided what may indeed be the most important tool for successfully living the "metabolic typing lifestyle." Nancy's hard won and heartfelt contribution to all of us in the form of the <u>Metabolic Typing® Cookbooks</u> is a natural expression of that rare, priceless combination of time, talent and experience, combined with a giving nature and a loving heart.

The world is rife with so-called experts. These days, anyone can write a book, self-publish it on the internet and with a little marketing savvy, appear authoritative. But the truth is that which lasts longest. And it is as true today as it has been since time immemorial, that expertise is possible only from the knowledge and understanding born from experience. Nancy Dale has an abundance of both.

Nancy has been one of the most active Certified Metabolic Typing® Advisors in the world over the last 5 years and her thriving, extremely successful practice with hundreds of enthusiastic, happy clients is testament to her expertise. Nancy's background as a successful, professional chef, combined with her extensive clinical experience with Metabolic Typing® makes her uniquely qualified to author these cookbooks. We are all fortunate to have them, myself included!

Read them. Use them. And enjoy the energy, well-being and good health that surely will ensue!

William L. Wolcott
Author, <u>The Metabolic Typing® Diet</u> (Doubleday, 2000)
Winthrop, Washington, December, 2009

Acknowledgement

This has been the most rewarding project I have ever worked on. This book along with the other five metabolic typing ® cookbooks has been a labor of love.

The bulk of the recipes were created from teaching my cooking classes throughout the years. It was not until 2009 that I actually fine-tuned the recipes to have only the ingredients for each particular type for each recipe- not an easy task when you consider each recipe must be created using only those ingredients.

A special thanks to Meg Fish for her amazing photography and her special artistic touch seen throughout the books; neither one of us had ever edited or created a book before so it was a pleasure to have someone so full of energy and enthusiasm to work with.

I would also like to acknowledge Bill Wolcott for his wonderful support and encouragement. Without him we would not have this incredible metabolic typing ® approach to health.

To all my students and clients who have tasted my recipes and to all of you who are about to try them; I hope you like them as much as I do.

Eating to live, not living to eat.

Nancy Dale

Introduction

These recipes are meant to be a starting point; adding more or less of any of the proteins, fats and carbohydrates until you feel satisfied. Experiment; this is how I created these recipes with the intent of customizing to fit your needs.

Most of the recipes are for multiple meals. I actually cook on Sunday for all week. I choose what recipes I am going to make and create a shopping list of ingredients a day or two prior to cooking. I involve everyone in the fun of choosing what they would like to eat. On the week-end I reserve a couple of hours to cook all of the meals for the upcoming week.

When the food has cooled, I divide each portion so that each person has the right amount to begin with.

It is a complete delight for me to walk into my kitchen at the end of a long day and open my refrigerator to any number of meals I have made that can be easily re-heated in the oven or on the stove top. In minutes we are sitting down to a great home cooked meal. This can also be very important if you have multiple Metabolic Types® in one family.

I generally steam different vegetables that can be eaten by all as well. When I am making poultry I try to have dark meat as well as breast meat.

Having multiple meals at your finger tips will help to keep everyone eating the right foods for their Metabolic Type ®.

- If you have food sensitivities omit the offending food that you have reactions to or substitute with another food from the same macronutrient group. Example: Instead of asparagus use cauliflower. Instead of salmon use halibut.

- If you have weight issues try to eat less at each meal by a mouthful or two. Wait twenty minutes and see if you are comfortable. This is what I call **"mindfully under eating"**.

- Eat sitting down at a table without distractions from the TV or computer. Never eat standing up or in your car.

- Do not eat if you are really stressed. Instead have a glass of water relax for a few minutes and wait until you have calmed down.

- Sweeteners such as stevia can be exchanged for xylitol, maple syrup, organic pure cane sugar or fruit juice, but use less of them and taste for sweetness, (less is better). You may substitute honey only in the dishes that do not require cooking, such as the yogurt or protein smoothies.

- Remember after each meal or snack you should feel satisfied, have great energy, have a sense of feeling renewed and restored. You should not have food cravings or a desire for more food. If you have any bad reactions such as feeling full, but still hungry or hyper, jittery you need to make sure you ate the right amount of protein, fats and carbohydrates for your type. An example of this might be at breakfast eating eggs makes you sluggish. Try having a protein smoothie and see if that makes you feel more energized. **This is what this whole process is about**. Learning exactly what fuel works in each body at each meal.   For additional help please contact your Metabolic Typing ® advisor to help you fine-tune this process.

Glycemic Index

Grains

Corn bread	110	Stoned wheat thins	67
Instant rice	91	Quick Oats	65
Corn chips	72	Basmati white rice	58
Millet	71	Whole wheat pita	57
Corn tortilla	70	White rice	56
Corn meal	68	Corn	55
Rye crackers	68	Oatmeal, old fashioned	48
Taco shell	68	Bulgur	48
Couscous	65	Barley	25

Bread

French baguette	95	Hamburger bun	61
Pretzels	81	Cheese pizza	60
Kaiser roll	73	Bran muffin	60
Bagel	72	Blueberry muffin	60
White bread	70	Pita	57
Melba toast	70	Sourdough	54
Whole wheat	69	Oat bran	54
Rye	65	Banana	47
Croissant	67	Pumpernickel	41

Pasta

Linguine	55	Vermicelli	35
Cheese Tortellini	50	Spaghetti	35
Macaroni	45	Fettuccini	32
Spaghetti	44	Spaghetti(protein enrich)	28
" " whole wheat	37		

Beverages

Gatorade	78	Grapefruit juice	51
Cranberry juice	68	Pineapple juice	48
Coca cola	63	Apple juice	41
Orange juice	55	Tomato juice	38

Dairy

Yogurt with fruit	36	Yogurt	14
Milk (fat free)	32	Whole milk	30
Cottage cheese	24		

Fruit

Watermelon	72	Orange	43
Pineapple	66	Grapes	43
Cantaloupe	65	Strawberries	40
Raisins	64	Apple	36
Apricot	31	Pear	36

Fruits, Cont.			
Papaya	60	Peaches	28
Banana	53	Plum	24
Kiwi	52	Grapefruit	25
Date	50	Cherries	22
Potato			
Potato	104	Mashed potato	73
Red potato	93	Potato chips	54
Instant mashed	83	Sweet potato	54
French fries	76	Yam	51
Legumes			
Pea soup	66	Lima beans	32
Split pea and ham	66	Chick peas	32
Black beans	54	Navy beans	31
Butter beans	36	Lentils	30
Black eyed peas	42	Kidneys	23
Garbanzo	34	Peanuts	13
Beans (string/green)	0		
Nuts			
Cashews	22	Macadamia	0
Almonds	0	Pecans	0
Brazil	0	Walnuts	0
Hazelnuts	0		
Vegetables			
Carrots	92	Eggplant	0
Beets	64	Snow peas	0
Tomato	15	Artichoke	0
Mushroom	0	Peppers	0
Broccoli	0	Asparagus	0
Cauliflower	0	Zucchini	0
Cabbage	0	Cucumber	0
Celery	0	Lettuce	0
Meat/Protein			
Beef	0	Lamb	0
Chicken	0	Pork	0
Eggs	0	Fish	0

Try to keep most of your choices below "40".

Facts on Fiber

What does fiber do? There are two types of fiber: insoluble (the kind found in vegetables, wheat and whole grains) and soluble (the kind found in fruits, oats, barley and legumes).

Insoluble fiber seems to fight cancer by binding to or diluting cancer-causing agents in the gut and speeding them through the colon.

Soluble fiber has its own part to play in keeping the body healthy: preventing heart disease. This kind of fiber forms a gel in the intestines that traps and ushers cholesterol out of the body. Soluble fiber can help reduce insulin levels, which in turn lowers triglycerides.

High fiber diets slow down the rate of digestion, which lowers both blood sugar levels and the insulin needed to transport that blood sugar into the cells.

Foods high in soluble fiber stay in your stomach longer creating a feeling of fullness that lasts longer so you eat less. Eating a diet high in soluble fiber will allow you to lose an average of 1/2 pound per week.

Food	Fiber (grams)
wheat-bran cereal (1/2 cup)	11
oatmeal (1 cup cooked)	4
brown rice (1 cup)	3.5
barley (1/2 cup cooked)	3
whole wheat bread	2
potato (baked with skin on)	5
carrots (1/2 cup cooked)	3
Brussels sprouts (1/2 cup cooked)	2.5
black-eyed peas (1/2 cups cooked)	8
black beans (1/2 cup cooked)	7.5
kidney beans (1/2 cup cooked)	6.5
lima beans (1/2 cup cooked)	6.5
apple (with skin on)	4
pear (with skin on)	4
raisins (2/3 cup seedless)	4
raspberries (1/2 cup)	4
orange (1 medium)	3.5

Boosting your fiber intake to the recommended 25-35 grams a day is good for your health. It can cause excess gas and be tough on your stomach. Here are some tips to ease the discomfort.

Go slowly. Increase your fiber by 5 grams per week.

Think small. Eat smaller portions of problematic foods such as beans and whole grains. Eat fruit that contain insoluble fiber which are easier to digest.

Emotional Eating

You are continually nourished by the world around you. When you close yourself to that nutrition, you feel the need to provide it yourself.

That is when food becomes magnetic. You do not have the capacity to provide yourself with the nourishment that you crave, and so eating becomes endless. **It is not the calories you seek, but contact with your soul (going home) and with the universe.** That is where true satisfaction exists, and is complete, nourishing and sustains life. No amount of chocolate, chips, salsa, or macaroni and cheese can substitute for this.

You can not receive too much nourishment from the universe any more than you can breathe too much air. When you do not have enough air, you gasp. When you do not have enough nourishment for your soul you seek substitution in food. You can eat too much food.

Eating more than you need is not necessarily a sign of a chemical imbalance or eating the wrong types of food. It is a sign that you are fundamentally out of balance. Until that correction is made, compulsive hunger will continue to remind you that you have inner work to do. It is a gift; gentle reminders to pay attention to what is going on in your world and make the corrections to create a healthy body, mind and spirit.

Dieting and exercise cannot reach the root of obsessive eating. Eating the right foods in the right amounts and exercising are prerequisites for physical health. However, illnesses are symptoms of deeper dynamics that bear directly on the purpose of your life and where you are accomplishing it.

Eating is Sacred. Every time you eat or drink anything, say to yourself, "Eating is sacred. I eat this food to nourish my body."

When you emotionally eat you deprive yourself from learning about your emotions. Next time you go for the cookie when you have had a **"bad"** day consider sitting down and reflecting on the events of the day and see what you can learn from this.

What is more worthy of your attention—a gift of knowledge about yourself or a cookie?

Green = Option #1 (eat either #1 or #2 foods)
Purple = Option #2 (eat either #1 or #2 foods)
Black = For variety (but emphasize 'Ideal' foods)
Italics = Caution (eat only rarely)

Protein

Beef
Buffalo
Elk
Heart
Kidney
Lamb
Liver
Pork (bacon, chops)
Rabbit
Venison
Wild game
Chicken (dark meat)
Duck
Goose
Grouse
Pheasant
Quail
Turkey
Abalone
Anchovy
Arctic Char
Caviar
Clam
Crab
Crayfish
Herring
Lobster
Mackerel
Mussel
Octopus
Oyster
Perch
Salmon
Sardine
Scallop
Shrimp
Squid
Trout
Tuna (dark)
Pork (ham)
Chicken (white meat)
Cornish hen
Ostrich
Turkey (white meat)
Bass (freshwater)
Bass (sea)
Cod
Flounder
Grouper

Protein, cont'd

Halibut
Mahi-mahi
Perch
Rockfish
Roughy
Snapper
Tuna
Turbot
Catfish
Pompano
Shark
Snail/Escargot
Whitefish

Vegetables

Arugula
Beet Greens
Cilantro
Dandelion Greens
Endive
Kale
Mustard
Swiss chard
Broccoli
Brussels Sprout
Cabbage
Cucumber
Pepper (hot, all colors)
Squash (winter)
Shallot
Tomato
Bamboo Shoots
Bok Choy
Daikon
Eggplant
Jicama
Kohlrabi
Peppers (bell, all colors)
Radish
Water chestnuts
Zucchini
Parsnip
Pumpkin
Potato
Rutabaga

Scallions
Onion
Squash (summer)
Collard greens
Lettuce (all)
Spinach
Turnip Greens
Watercress
Asparagus
Cauliflower
Celery
Mushroom
Avocado
Green Beans
Jerusalem Artichoke
Olives (all)
Okra
Turnip
Artichoke
Beet
Carrots
Corn
Green Peas
Sweet peas
Parsley
Radicchio
Sprouts
Garlic
Ginger Root
Fennel
Sweet Potato

Grains

Cornmeal
Rice (basmati)
Rice (brown)
Wheat
Wild rice
Millet
Amaranth
Barley
Buckwheat
Kamut
Oat
Quinoa
Rye
Spelt
Triticale

15

| **Fruits** | **Dairy** | **Condiments, Spices** |

Fruits

Apple
Apricot
Banana
Blackberry
Blueberry
Boysenberry
Cantaloupe
Casaba melon
Cherry
Coconut
Cranberry
Elderberry
Gooseberry
Grape
Guava
Honeydew melon
Kiwifruit
Kumquat
Loganberry
Mango
Nectarine
Papaya
Peach
Pear (just ripe)
Persimmon
Pineapple
Plum
Pomegranate
Raspberry
Rhubarb
Strawberry
Watermelon
Grapefruit
Lime
Orange
Lemon
Tangerine
Currant (dried)
Date, prune, raisin
Fig

Dairy

Blue cheese
Brie
Camembert
Cheddar
Colby
Cream cheese
Edam
Goat cheese
Gouda
Gruyere
Monterey Jack
Muenster
Parmesan
Provolone
Romano
Roquefort
Swiss
Buttermilk
Cottage Cheese
Milk (whole)
Cream
Feta
Goat milk
Kefir
Mozzarella
Neufchatel
Ricotta
Sour cream
Whey
Yogurt (full fat)
Eggs, chicken
Eggs, duck

Nuts & Seeds

Brazil Nuts
Walnuts
Filbert
Hazelnut
Flax
Hickory nuts
Macadamia nuts
Peanuts
Pecans
Pumpkin seeds
Almonds
Cashews
Chestnuts
Pine Nuts
Pistachios
Poppy Seeds
Sesame Seeds
Sunflower Seeds

Condiments, Spices

Anise
Basil
Bay leaf
Caraway
Chervil
Chive
Dill weed
Fennel seed
Fenugreek
Garlic powder
Marjoram
Mustard seed
Parsley
Cumin
Ginger
Nutmeg
Pepper (black)
Chocolate
Hot sauce
Honey
Mustard
Sea salt
Wasabi
Vinegar (apple, balsamic, rice)
Rosemary
Sage
Savory
Spearmint
Tarragon
Thyme
Cardamom
Cayenne
Chili powder
Cinnamon
Clove
Oregano
Coriander
Curry powder
Mace
Paprika
Saffron
Carob
Horseradish
Ketchup
Maple syrup
Soy sauce
Vanilla
Yeast

<u>**Oils & Fats**</u>

Butter (salted)
Butter (unsalted)
Coconut oil
Flax oil
Ghee
Olive oil
Palm oil
Almond oil
Walnut oil
Sesame oil
Sunflower oil
Safflower oil
Hemp oil
Peanut oil

The Balanced Type Diet

The balanced type diet falls between the carbohydrate type and the protein type diet blending the two. The mix type does have some tendencies in common:

Appetite varies-Some are hungry at mealtime but rarely get hungry in-between meals, while others have a ravenous appetite and then skip meals at other times.

Cravings-If mixed type do not eat balance they can develop sweet cravings. Making sure to eat Metabolic Type ® meals from the same option color will help this.

Weight Control-Typically mixed types do not have a weight problem if they stick with their MT diet plan making sure they eat balance from all three macronutrients, proteins, fats and carbohydrates.

- **The mix type needs balance** from both the carbohydrate low purine foods and the high purine foods from the protein type.
- **Eat protein at every meal.** Making sure that even snacks have protein will help to keep your blood sugar stable as well as keep you from cravings.
- **Avoid alcohol and caffeine.** Alcohol is a plain sugar and is a poison to the body. Caffeine stimulates and eventually exhausts the body.
- **Sugar and fruit juices** should be avoided as they cause an insulin surge that rapidly lowers blood sugars and increases fat storage.
- **Gluten and high starch** carbohydrates should be avoided as they are hard to digest and they can cause acid reflux as well as weight gain.

Food Menu's for #3-A, Balanced

Breakfast

Protein smoothie or
Egg Frittata with fruit or a Apple Coconut muffin or
Almond meal pancakes with eggs or
Yogurt with fruit and nuts or
Salmon Omelet with zucchini muffin

Lunch

Grilled Salmon on an Arugula Salad with Tomatoes or
Black Bean Chili or
Santa Barbara Salad with a zucchini muffin or
Enchiladas with Sliced Tomatoes and Arugula Salad or
Chicken and Spinach Soup with a Pear Almond Green Salad

Dinner

Turkey Meatloaf with Quinoa corn salad or
Rolled Chicken Stuffed Vegetables Papaya and Walnut Salad or
Baked fish with Mashed Cauliflower "Potatoes" or
Bacon Wrapped Pork Tenderloin with Sautéed Vegetables or
Salmon Cakes with Mango Salsa or
Greek Stuffed Steak with Steamed broccoli

Snacks

2 T. almond butter with ½ apple or pear
3-5 ounces yogurt with ½ cup fruit
¼ cup raw unsalted organic peanuts
½ banana with peanut butter
Celery and carrots with ranch dressing

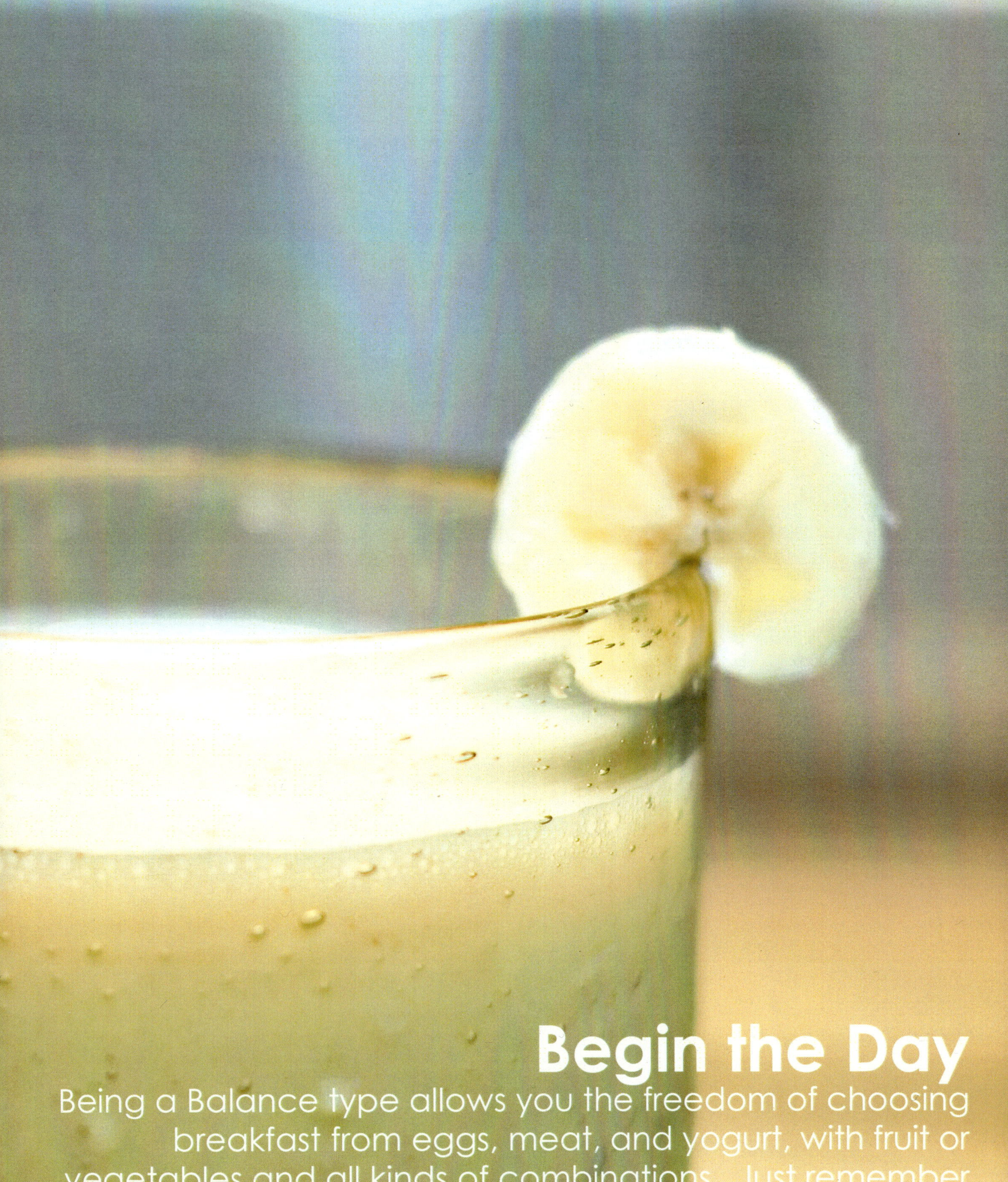

Begin the Day
Being a Balance type allows you the freedom of choosing
breakfast from eggs, meat, and yogurt, with fruit or
vegetables and all kinds of combinations. Just remember
to eat from all three macronutrients, protein, fat and
carbohydrates at each meal.

Almond Pancakes

(Calories per pancake: 125, 6 g protein, 8 g fat, 6 g carbohydrates)

Serves 2-4

| 1 | Mix ingredients together and cook as you would other pancakes.

They will not bubble, so turn when side becomes light brown. | 1 C. almond meal
2 eggs, lightly beaten
¼ C. water
¼ C. chopped apples
2 T. coconut oil
1 T. stevia
½ t. cinnamon
¼ t. sea salt |
| 2 | Serve with pat of butter and chopped almonds and sliced apples. | butter
almonds
apple |

Tip: You must use medium high heat to cook through and brown. Be sure and add some protein (eggs or sausage or yogurt) along with this to complete the meal.

Asparagus and Mushrooms over Eggs
(Calories: 200, 8 g protein, 12 g fat, 10 g carbohydrates)

Serves 2-4

1	Slice asparagus into ½ inch pieces and heat in oil adding mushrooms sautéing until tender crisp about 8 minutes.	1 lb. asparagus, trimmed 1 T. olive oil ½ lb. mushrooms, trimmed
2	Add more oil and sauté onions and cook for 8 minutes or until soft.	2 T. olive oil ½ onion, chopped fine
3	Scramble or poach eggs and place one or two on each plate. Place mixture over eggs and sprinkle with cheese. Serve immediately.	4-6 eggs ¼ C. mozzarella, grated ¼ t. sea salt ¼ t. pepper

Protein Smoothies

Serves one each recipe: In blender (may add raw egg)

1	**Basic Berry**- Combine milk, fruit and protein powder in blender. May use sunflower seeds if desired for extra fiber.	1-1½ C. organic milk, rice or almond milk 1 C. frozen berries 1 scoop whey, Goatein, hemp, egg white or rice protein powder 1 T. sunflower seeds(optional)
2	**Creamy Monkey**- Mix milk, protein powder, peanut or almond butter and banana; blend.	1-1½ C. organic milk, rice or almond milk 1 scoop hemp, egg white or rice protein powder 1 T. peanut butter ½ frozen banana
3	**Reese's Pieces**- Same ingredients as creamy monkey but add organic cocoa powder.	Use 1 T. cocoa powder to above recipe for Creamy monkey.
4	**Tropical Delight**-Combine milk, banana, pineapple, mango with protein powder; blend until smooth. May use flax seeds if needed for more fiber.	1-1½ C. organic milk, rice or almond milk ½ frozen banana ¼ C. frozen pineapple ¼ C. frozen mango 1 scoop hemp or rice protein powders 1 T. ground flax seeds*
5	**Raspberry Delight**-Blend milk, protein powder, raspberries with cocoa until smooth. May use sunflower seeds.	1-1½ C. organic milk, rice or almond milk 1 scoop whey, hemp, Goatein , egg white or rice protein powder ½ C. frozen raspberries 1 T. cocoa 1 T. sunflower seeds(optional)

*May use ground flax seed or flax seed oil.

Tip: Choose the protein powder that works best with your food option.

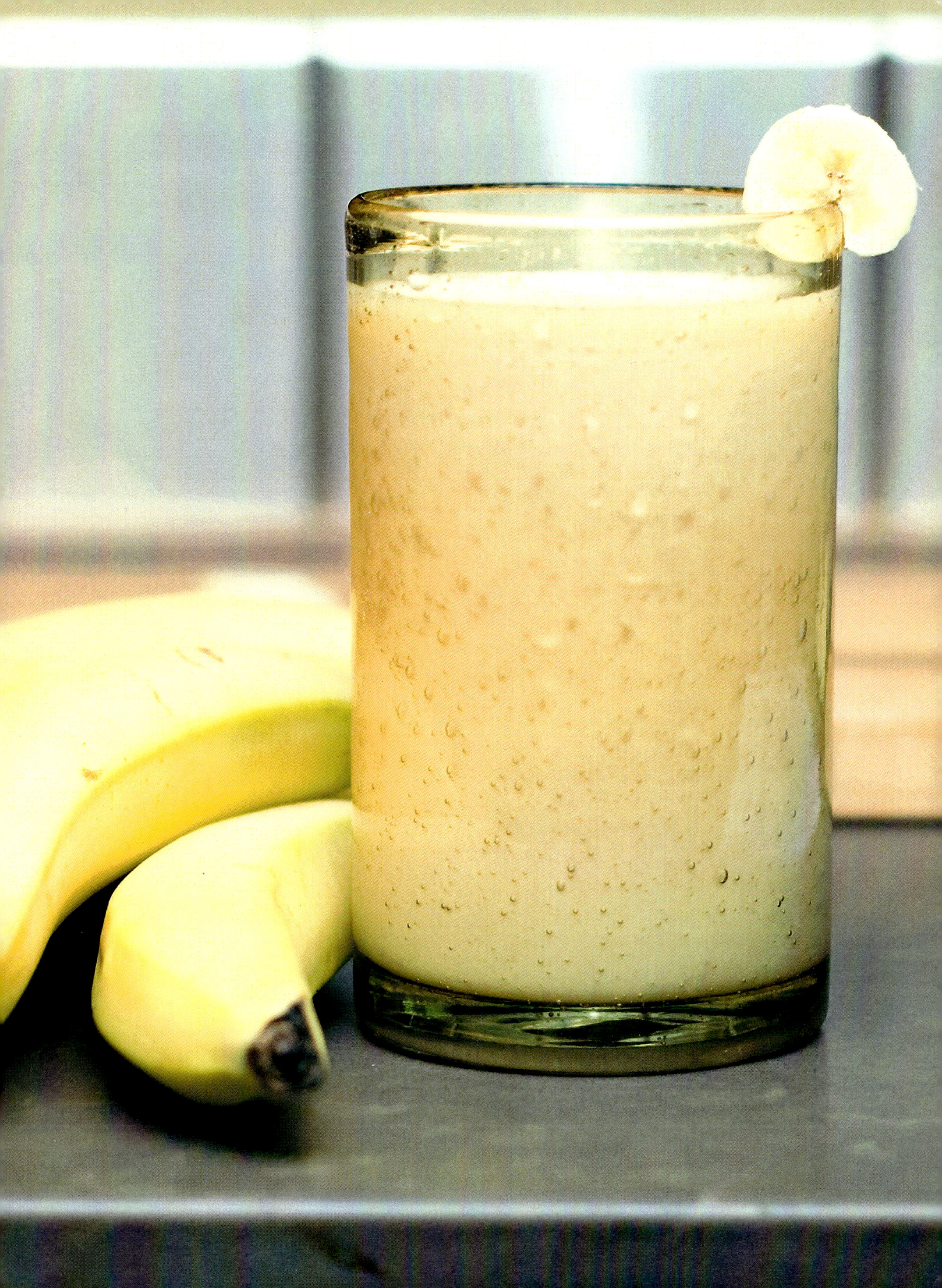

Mini Mushroom and Sausage Quiches
(Calories per two muffins: 225, 18 g protein, 13 g fat, 10 g carbohydrates)

Makes 10-12 small muffins

1	Preheat oven to 325° F	
2	Heat skillet over medium flame. Add sausage and cook 6-8 minutes. Drain and transfer to a bowl and let cool 5 minutes	8 oz. pork sausage, removed from casing and crumbled into small pieces
3	Add oil to the skillet and cook mushrooms stirring often until golden brown about 5-7 minutes. Transfer to the sausage bowl and let cool 5 minutes. Stir in spinach, feta and pepper.	1-2 t. olive oil 8 oz. mushrooms, sliced ½ C. spinach, cooked and drained ¼ C. goat feta cheese ½ t. black pepper
4	Whisk in a bowl the eggs and milk until frothy. Divide the egg mixture evenly among the oiled and papered muffin cups. Place a heaping tablespoon of the sausage mixture into each cup.	8 organic free-range eggs 1 C. organic whole milk foil muffin liners 1 T. olive oil
5	Bake until the tops are just beginning to brown, about 25 minutes.	
6	Individually wrap in plastic for up to 3 days or freeze.	makes 10-12 small muffins

Sausage Mushroom Spinach Frittata
(Calories: 350, 35 g protein, 12 g fat 25 g carbohydrates)

Serves 6

1	Preheat oven to 400° F	
2	Oil and sprinkle pie or quiche pan with almond meal; set aside.	1 T. olive oil or coconut oil ¼ C. almond meal(may substitute bread crumbs)
3	In a skillet melt butter and add mushrooms cooking 3-4 minutes on medium flame. Slice the sausages and add to mushrooms and cook 2-3 minutes.	1-2 T. raw organic butter 4 oz. mushrooms, sliced 8-12 oz. pork sausages
4	Steam the spinach leaves 2-3 minutes and squeeze out any moisture. Add to mushroom mixture.	4-6 oz. of organic spinach leaves
5	Mix together in a bowl. Beat until well mixed.	¼ C. organic whole milk 10-12 organic free-range eggs ¼ t. sea salt ¼ t. pepper
6	Place mushroom mixture in pan with almond meal and top with feta cheese.	4 oz. feta cheese
7	Pour egg mixture over all.	
8	Bake for 30 minutes.	

Salmon Omelet

(Calories: 250, 24 g protein, 13 g fat, 8 g carbohydrates)

Serves 2, may be doubled for 4

1	Preheat oven to 350° F	
2	Separate egg yolks and lightly beat, set side. Combine the 4 egg whites in a small mixing bowl and beat until light and fluffy. Add egg yolks and salt and pepper.	2 large eggs and 2 egg whites ¼ t. sea salt ¼ t. pepper
3	Lightly oil an oven proof skillet and place over medium heat. Spread the egg mixture in the pan and cook for 3-5 minutes until the bottom is light brown.	1 T. coconut oil or butter
4	Place the skillet in the hot oven on the middle rack and bake 3 minutes. Dot with goat cheese, salmon and tomatoes and parsley and bake 1 more minute.	3 oz. goat cheese 3 oz. smoked salmon (or left over salmon) 4 cherry tomatoes split in half
5	To serve fold the omelet in half.	

Tip: This recipe needs fruit or vegetables to complete the meal.

Apple Coconut Flour Nut Muffins
(Calories: 184, 12 g protein, 8 g fat, 16 g carbohydrates)

Makes 12 muffins

1	Preheat oven to 350° F	
2	Mix coconut flour and baking powder in a separate bowl, set aside.	1 C. coconut flour* 1 t. baking powder
3	In a mixing bowl, beat eggs gradually…. Add milk, stevia, coconut oil, butter, vanilla and salt.	6 organic free range eggs 2 T. organic milk 1 T. stevia (substitute ¼ C. maple syrup) 2 T. coconut oil* (warmed to liquid) 2 T. organic butter ½ t. vanilla 1/8 t. sea salt
4	Add the apple to the egg mixture. Continue mixing and slowly add the flour mixture and sunflower seeds and mix until blended.	1 large apple, grated ½ C. sunflower pieces
5	Oil and fill muffin cups with batter.	
6	Bake for 20 minutes.	

*Purchase at www.tropicaltraditions.com

Zucchini Muffins

(Calories: 170, 7 g protein, 14 g fat, 2 g carbohydrates)

Makes 18 small muffins

1	Preheat oven to 350° F	
2	Grate. Set aside.	3 C. zucchini
3	Chop. Set aside.	1 C. walnuts
4	Sift into a bowl... ... and then add the grated zucchini and chopped walnuts	2 C. whole wheat flour ½ C. hemp or eggwhite protein powder 1 t. baking soda 2 t. cinnamon 1 t. ground ginger 1 t. ground nutmeg ¼ t. ground cloves ¼ t. salt
5	Mix together in another bowl.	3 eggs, slightly whipped ¼ C. maple syrup 1 t. vanilla 1/3 C. coconut oil ¼ C. pineapple juice
6	Pour wet mixture into dry mixture and mix well (You may need a little extra pineapple juice to make a soft batter).	
7	Spoon into a small muffin tin.	Bake for 20-25 minutes.

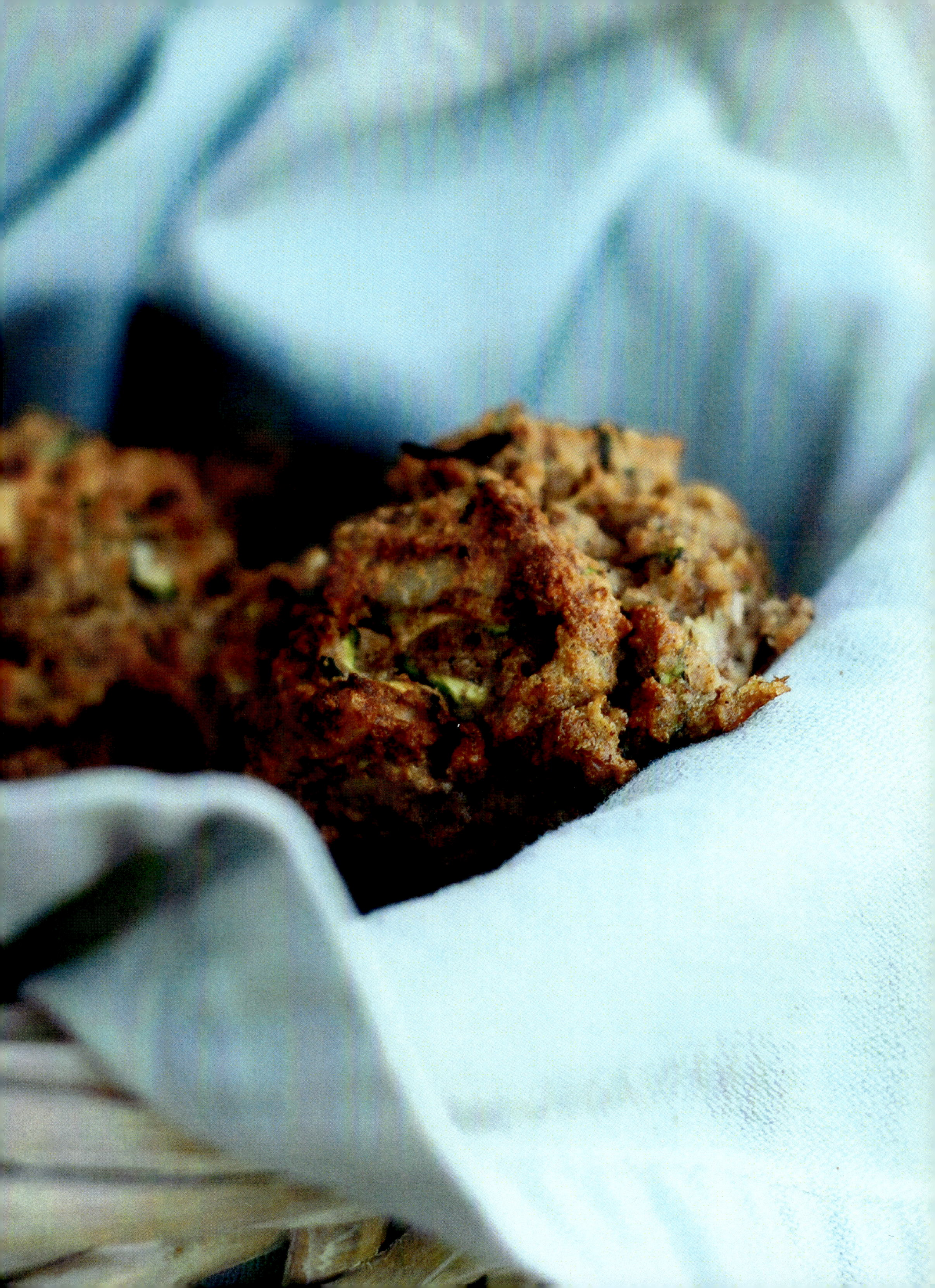

Santa Barbara Shrimp Salad Pg 38

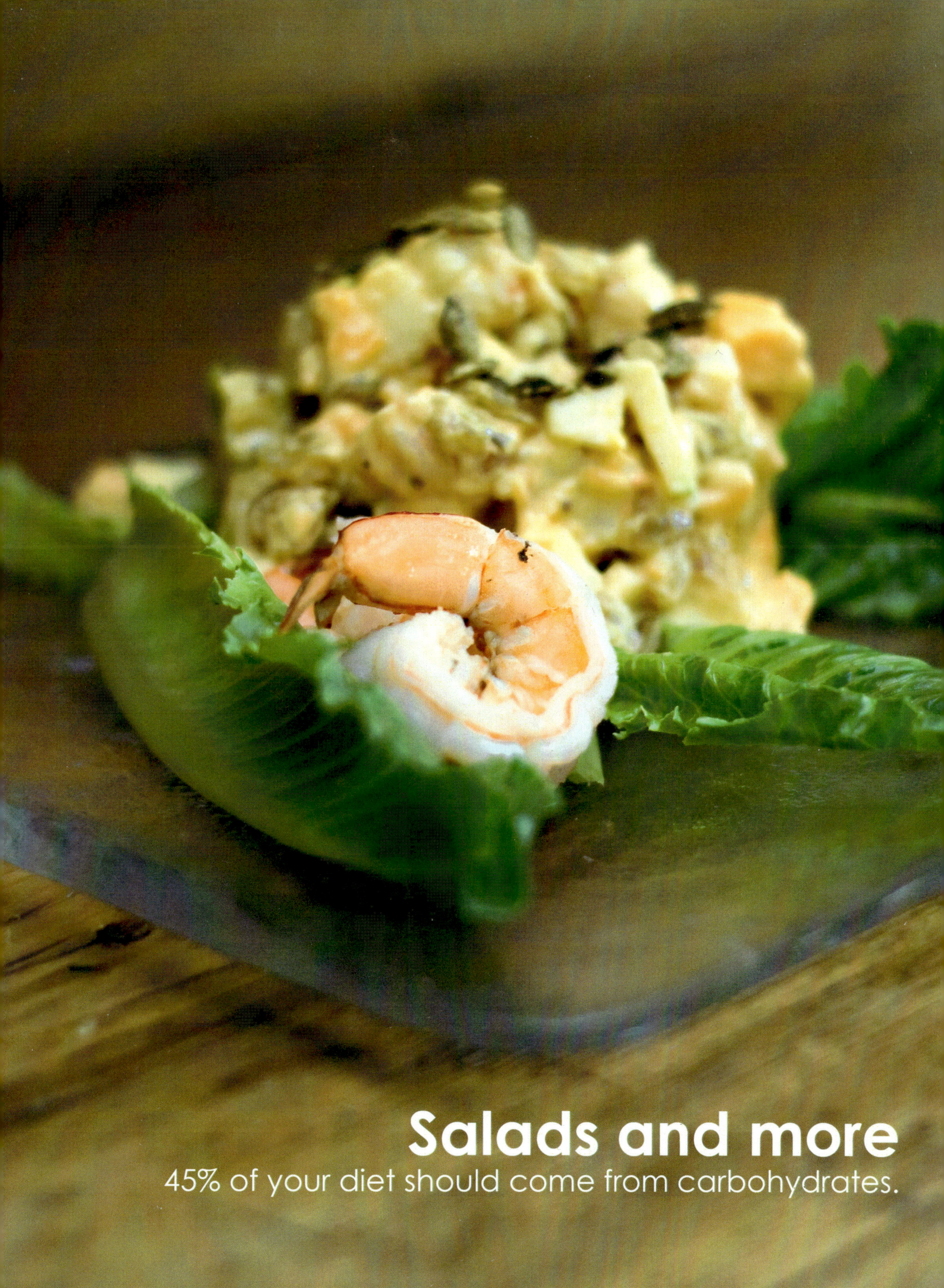
Salads and more
45% of your diet should come from carbohydrates.

Fresh Fig Salad with Toasted Pine Nuts
(Calories: 280, 8 g protein, 16 g fat, 24 g carbohydrates)

Serves 4-6

1	Clean and wipe the figs gently and cut in half. Wash the greens. Arrange 4-5 figs on each plate on top of the greens.	24 fresh black figs, medium size (can use dried) 4 oz. organic baby green lettuce mix
2	Crumble and sprinkle the feta cheese over the figs. Toast the pine nuts and scatter on top.	6 oz. feta goat cheese ½ C. pine nuts
3	Place vinegar and salt and pepper in a screw top jar and shake until salt dissolves. Add mustard and walnut oil; shake until emulsified.	1 T. balsamic vinegar ¼ t. sea salt ¼ t. pepper 1 t. Dijon mustard 6 T. walnut oil
4	Drizzle vinaigrette over fig salad and serve.	

Tip: This makes a great salad that needs a protein like Chicken Crusted in Almonds or Bacon-Wrapped Pork Tenderloin to make a balanced meal.

Papaya and Walnut Green Salad

(Calories: 250, 20 g protein, 8 g fat, 16 g carbohydrates)

Serves 4

1	Blend together until emulsified.	4 T. walnut oil (may use olive oil) 4 T. balsamic vinegar ¼ t. sea salt ¼ t. pepper
2	Wash and combine greens in a large bowl and toss the crumbled gorgonzola cheese on the greens.	12 oz. organic greens 2 oz. gorgonzola cheese
3	Slice the papaya and shallots and add to the greens.	1 organic papaya 2 shallots
4	Toast the walnuts and add to salad.	¼ C. walnuts
5	Drizzle the vinaigrette over salad and serve.	

Tip: Combine this with Beef Kabobs and enjoy.

Cold Asparagus with Sesame-ginger Vinaigrette
(Calories: 150, 2 g protein, 11 g fat, 10 g carbohydrates)

Serves 4

1	Mix dressing together and chill.	1 clove garlic, minced 2 T. orange juice 2 T. olive oil ¼ t. red chili flakes 1 t. grated fresh ginger 2 t. Braggs Liquid Aminos 1/8 t. stevia ¼ t. toasted sesame oil
2	On a bed of spinach leaves place chilled cooked asparagus and pour dressing on top.	1 lb. asparagus, trimmed, steamed and chilled 1 bunch of fresh cleaned spinach leaves

Tip: This works well with Rolled Chicken Stuffed with Vegetables.

Tuna Dip

(Calories 250, 10 g protein, 15 g fat, 30 g carbohydrates)

Serves 4

1	Blend together tuna, green onion and celery in a food processor or blender (do not puree).	1 12 ½ oz. can light tuna, water packed, drained. 1 green onion 1 small celery stalk
2	Blend in mayonnaise, lemon juice and salt and pepper.	¼ C. mayonnaise 1 T. lemon juice ¼ t. sea salt ¼ t. pepper
3	Blend to desired consistency and sprinkle with parsley.	¼ C. parsley leaves
4	Fill ½ avocado with tuna mixture and place on a bed of lettuce.	2 avocado 4 C. salad greens

Tip: Serve this for a light lunch or appetizer.

Santa Barbara Shrimp Salad
(Calories: 354, 23 g protein, 14 g fat, 34 g carbohydrates)

Serves 4

1	Mix ingredients in a small bowl. Cover and chill.	½ C. mayonnaise 1 T. curry powder 1 T. lime juice 1 t. fresh ginger, minced
2	Heat sake with raisins in a small pot; let stand for 30 minutes.	½ C. sake(optional may use warm water) ½ C. golden raisins
3	Bring sake to a boil in a skillet: add shrimp, cover and reduce heat and cook 2 minutes. Remove from heat; drain.	¼ C. sake 1 lb. wild caught shrimp, peeled and deveined*
4	Dice the pineapple and mango into ½ inch pieces.	1½ C. pineapple, fresh 4 C. mango
5	Combine mayonnaise mixture, drunken raisins, shrimp, pineapple and mango.	
6	Toss in pumpkin seeds.	6 T. pumpkin seeds
7	Divide salad greens into 4 plates Serve salad over greens.	8 C. organic arugula salad greens

*Can be purchased at www.great-alaskan-seafood.com

Tip: This salad keeps well and tastes even better the next day. Keep in a tight container and place on arugula greens right before serving.

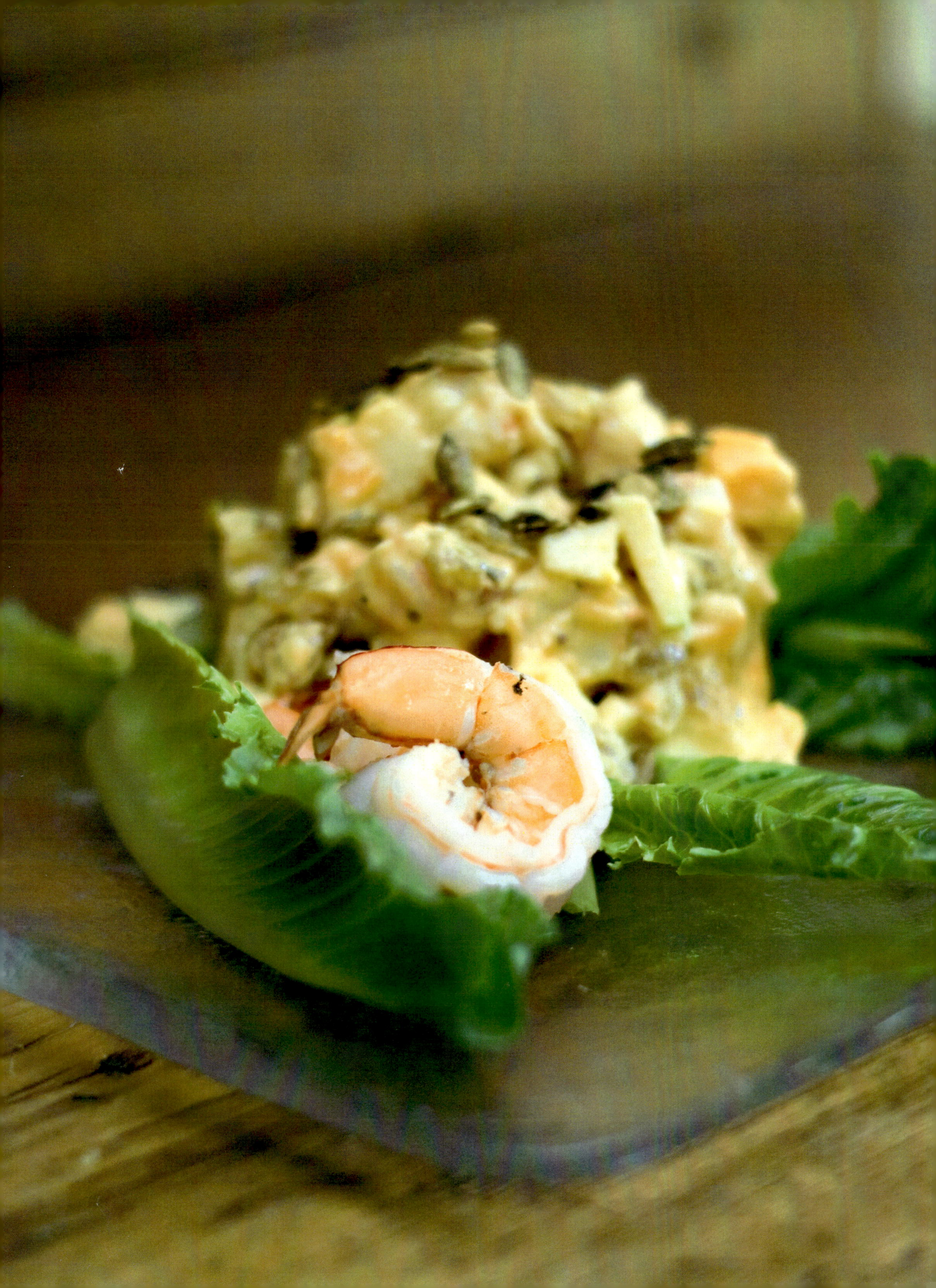

Lentil Salad
(1/2 C. serving 200 calories, 12 g protein, 4 g fat, 29 g carbohydrates)

Serves 4-6

1	Sort through and wash the lentils. In a pot cover the lentils with water. Bring to a boil, add bay leaf, cover and lower heat to a simmer, stirring occasionally and cook for 20-25 minutes until done. Drain in a colander.	1 ½ C. lentils 1 bay leaf
2	Soak currants in hot water for approximately 15 minutes, drain.	¼ C. currants
3	In a medium pan sauté onion in oil until soft about 5 minutes. Chop carrot and add to onion in pan for 2 minutes.	2 T. olive oil ½ C. onion 1 medium carrot
4	Place drained lentils in with the onion mixture and toss in the pine nuts and soy sauce.	¼ C. pine nuts 1 T. tamari wheat free soy sauce
5	Serve warm or at room temperature.	

Quinoa Corn Salad

(1 cup serving: Calories: 235, 10 g protein, 4 g fat, 40 g carbohydrates)

Serves 4

1	Bring the water to a light boil in a medium saucepan. Rinse quinoa in cold water to make sure it is clean; add to the water simmer twenty minutes. If there is extra liquid drain quinoa and place in a bowl.	1 C. quinoa 2 C. water
2	Combine corn, scallions and parsley with quinoa and chill.	½ C. frozen corn 2 scallions, chopped 1 T. parsley leaves
3	Divide greens and place on four salad plates.	14 oz. package of baby greens, rinsed
4	Combine olive oil. Salt and pepper and lime juice and shake until emulsified. Pour over quinoa mixture.	1-2 T. olive oil ¼ t. sea salt ¼ t. pepper juice of one organic lime
5	Divide quinoa and place over each bed of lettuce. Sprinkle seeds over and serve.	2 T. sunflower seeds

Tip: To make this a complete meal, serve with a halibut fillet or a grilled chicken breast. Or try tossing ¼ lb. cooked medium shrimp into the salad.

Black Bean and Corn Salad
(Calories: 170, 12 g protein, 5 g fat, 19 g carbohydrates)

Serves 4-6

1	Defrost the corn and place in a bowl. Drain the black beans and add to the bowl.	2 C. organic frozen corn 4 C. organic black beans (2 can 14.5 ounces)
2	Dice the celery and onion and add to the bowl.	1 stalk celery ½ red onion
3	Chop the parsley, using the leaves only.	½ C. parsley
4	In a small bowl whisk together olive oil, lime juice, garlic and salt and pepper.	¼ C. olive oil juice of one lime 1 garlic, minced ¼ t. sea salt ¼ t. pepper
5	Pour olive oil mixture over corn and beans and toss.	
6	Serve at room temperature or chill.	
7	May be refrigerated for 4 days.	

Tip: To create a balanced meal; serve with Bacon-Wrapped Pork or Grilled Chicken breast and a green salad.

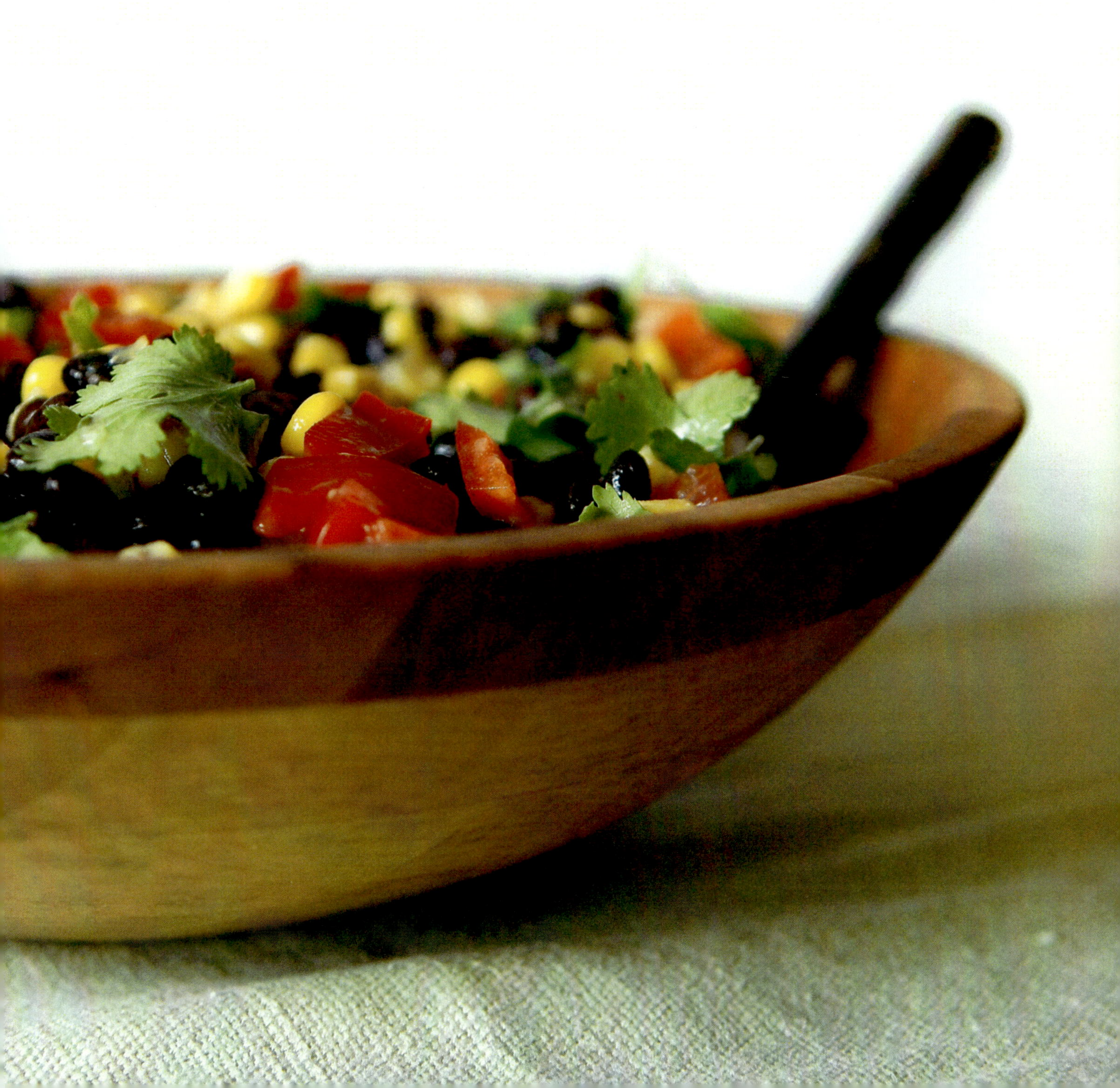

Artichoke and Ripe Olive Tuna Salad on Avocado
(Calories: 370, 20 g protein, 24 g fat, 12 g carbohydrates)

Serves 5

1	Combine ingredients in a bowl.	1-12 oz. can or 2-6 oz. cans light tuna in water 1 C. chopped artichoke hearts ½ C. chopped olives ¼ C. mayonnaise 2 t. lemon juice 1½ t. chopped fresh oregano or ½ t. dried ¼ t. sea salt ¼ t. pepper
2	Place Boston lettuce on salad plate with ¼ avocado. Place 1/5 of the tuna salad (¾ cup) on each avocado. Serve immediately.	5 Boston lettuce leaves 2-3 avocados, peeled and quartered

Tip: This is a very high fat salad add more lettuce to make it more balanced and eat with a cup of Split Pea and Ham Soup.

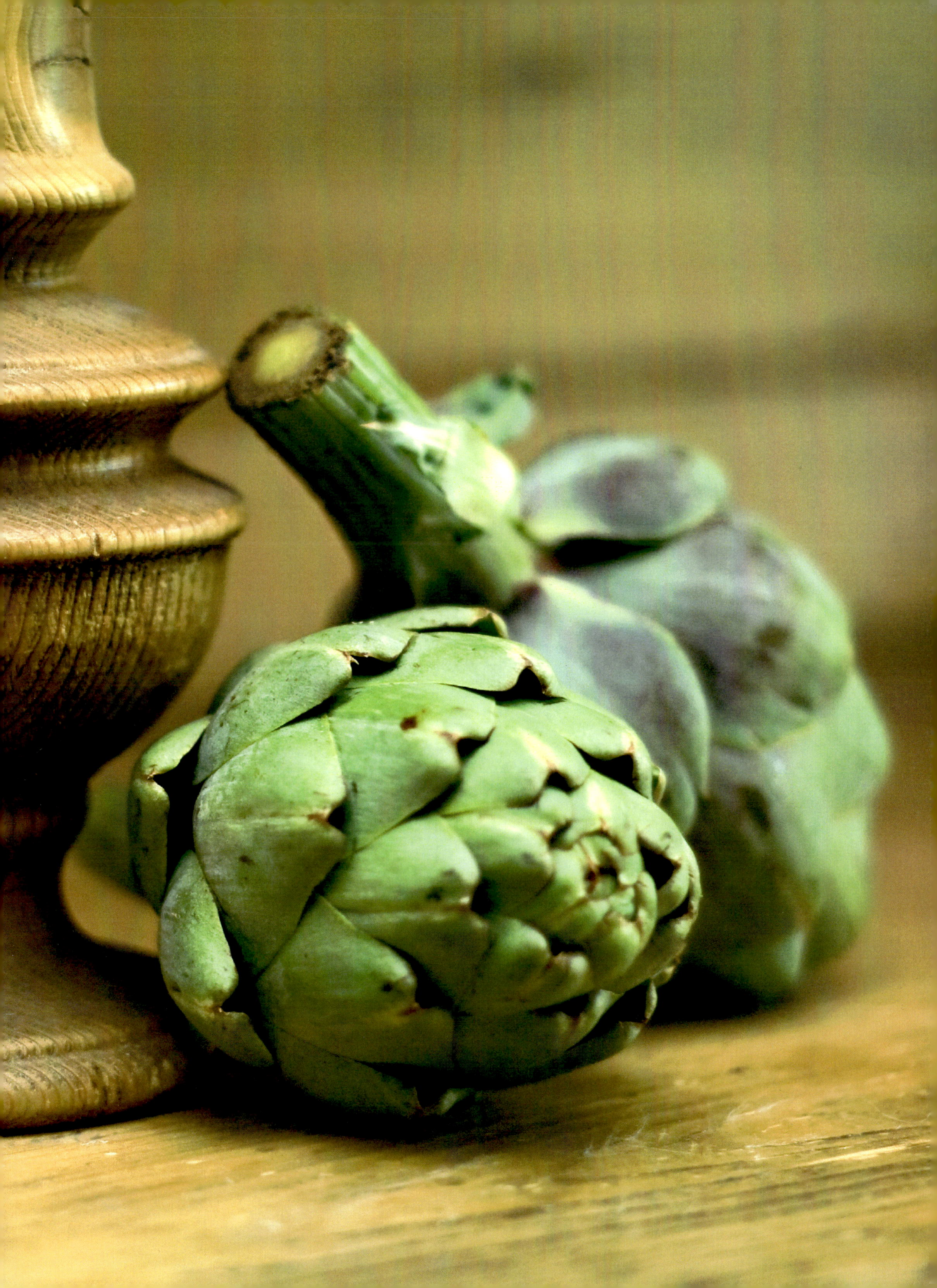

Chicken and Spinach Soup with Fresh Pesto Pg 54

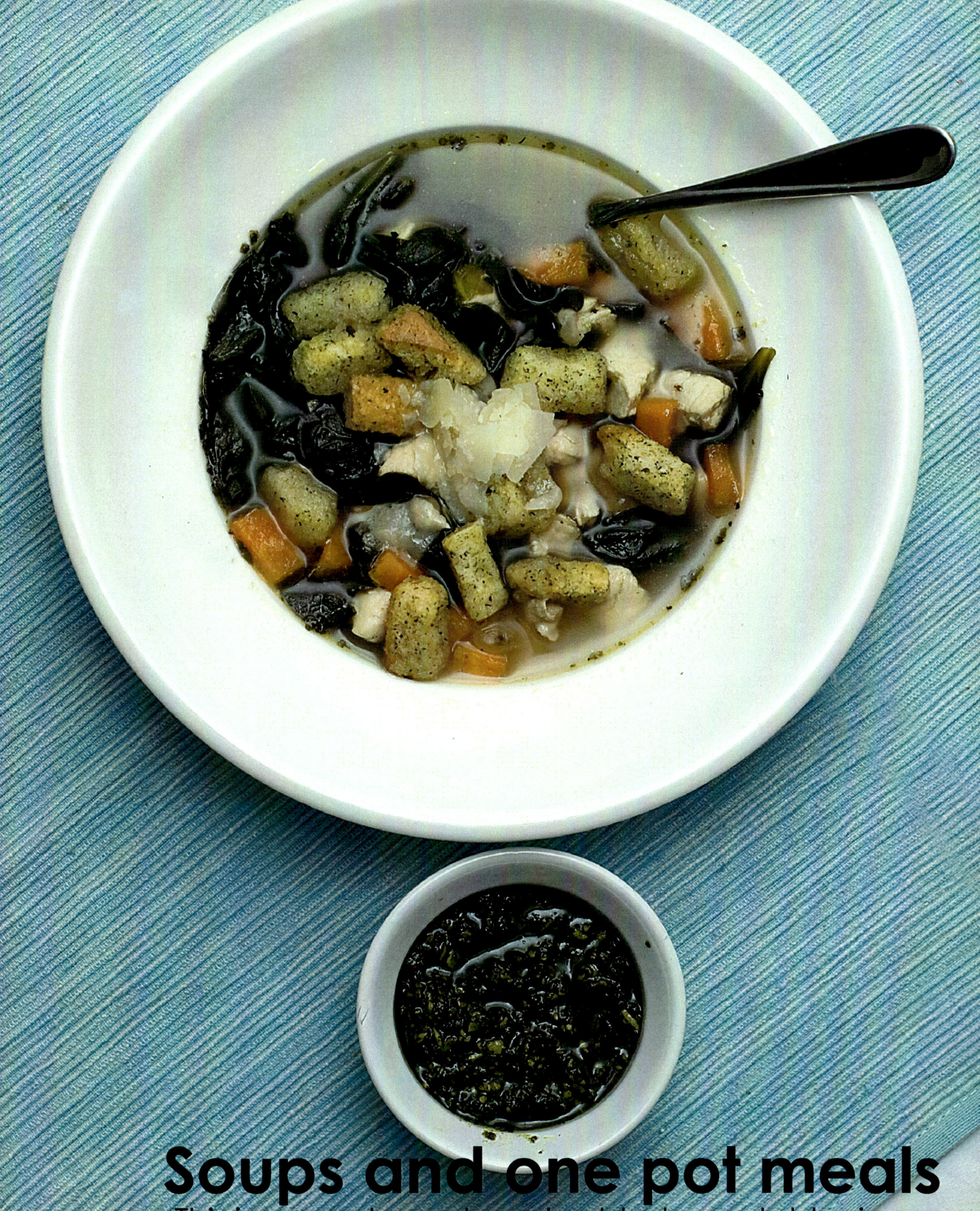

Soups and one pot meals

This is a great way to get added vegetables in our meals. Be sure and add protein to the meal if the recipe does not call for it.

Vegetable Broth #2

1	In a soup pan place cut up vegetables in 1 quart of filtered water and bring to a boil. Reduce and simmer about 6-8 minutes.	1 qt. filtered water 8 oz. green beans 2-4 stalks celery ½ bunch spinach leaves 4 oz. parsley
2	Puree in blender adding olive oil or butter, tamari, salt and pepper and cream.	1-2 T. olive oil or raw butter 1 T. Bragg's Aminos or tamari soy sauce ¼ t. sea salt ¼ t. pepper ¼ C. raw organic cream or milk
3	Place in air tight container; may be stored in refrigerator for 2-3 days.	

Tip: I make this and sip on it throughout the day for extra energy and to get my vegetables in.

Chicken Bone Broth

1	Place bones in a large pot and cover with water and add the vinegar. Let stand for one hour.	1 free range organic chicken, bones only 2 qts. filtered water 2 T. apple cider vinegar
2	Bring the pot to a simmering low boil and remove any foam scum that appears on the top of the water. Continue simmering on low boil for 24 hours.	
3	Remove bones and place in a container. Use or freeze for later use.	

Lentil Vegetable Soup
(Calories: 230, 17 g protein, 7 g fat, 25 g carbohydrates)

Serves 6-8

1	Heat oil in a large Dutch oven or stockpot over medium heat. Add onions, celery, carrots and bay leaves; sauté for 10 minutes.	1 T. olive oil 1 1/3 C. onions, chopped fine 1/3 C. celery, diced 1/3 C. carrots, diced 2 bay leaves
2	To the pot add salt and garlic and sauté another minute.	1 t. sea salt 2 garlic cloves, minced
3	Add the water and lentils; bring to a boil, partially cover and reduce heat, simmering for 25 minutes.	6 C. filtered water 1 C. dried dark green lentils
4	Stir in the chopped spinach, parsley, vinegar, mustard and pepper and cook on medium for 15 minutes.	6 C. spinach 1/3 C. chopped parsley 2 t. red wine vinegar 2 t. Dijon mustard ¼ t. black pepper
5	Discard the bay leaves. Ladle soup into bowls and top with cheese if desired.	3 oz. mozzarella cheese, grated
6	May add turkey to soup to make this a high protein soup.	6-8 oz. left over turkey (optional)

Tip: This makes a great lunch soup served with a green salad or muffin.

Tom Ka Kai (Chicken Soup)
(Calories: 219, 15 g protein, 7 g fat, 24 g carbohydrates)

Serves 4-6

1	Bring to a boil in a medium pot.	3 ½ C. coconut milk 2 C. chicken broth
2	Add to pot and lower heat to medium and simmer for 20 minutes.	1 *red chili (open with a knife) 4 stems of lemon grass, 1 inch pieces 1 inch ginger, peeled and sliced ¼ t. black pepper 6 lime leaves (optional)
3	Add to the pot and simmer another 10 minutes or until the chicken is done. Remove ginger, lemon grass and red chile from soup.	3 organic chicken breast, boned and skinned, cut into thin strips 2 oz. shitake mushrooms, sliced
4	Add scallions, lime and sea salt.	2 scallions, chopped ¼ C. lime juice Pinch of sea salt
5	Ladle into bowls and garnish with parsley.	1 T. parsley, leaves only

Tip: *Red chili is not this option, but it is removed and only used for flavor.
This makes a beautiful soup served with the Fresh Fig with Toasted Pine Nuts Salad or a green salad or your choice.

South of the Border Soup
(Calories: 324, 18 g protein, 8 g fat, 45 g carbohydrates)

Serves 4-6

1	In a soup pot bring broth to a boil; dice chicken and simmer covered for 10 minutes.	1 qt. chicken broth 4-6 chicken thighs, boneless, skinless
2	Add brown rice, zucchini, red pepper and green chilies; cook for 8 minutes.	½ C. brown rice, cooked 3 C. zucchini, diced 1½ C. red pepper, diced 1 4 oz. can green chilies, chopped
3	Add salsa and cook 2 minute more.	1 C. salsa
4	Pour into individual bowls and top with corn chips and shredded cheese. Serve with a wedge of lime.	¼ C. raw cheddar cheese ½ C. corn chips, crushed 1 lime, wedged

Tip: This is one of my favorite soups. It is easy to make and it tastes even better the next day.

Mushroom Barley Soup

(Calories: 300, 18 g protein, 10 g fat, 35 g carbohydrates)

Serves 6-8

1	In a large pot add oil and butter; sauté onion, celery, mushrooms for 5 minutes; Add garlic and tamari sauce and basil and cook 1 minute.	1 T. olive oil 2 T. raw butter 2 C. onions, diced 2 C. celery, diced 1 lb. mushrooms, sliced 2 cloves garlic, minced ¼ C. tamari wheat free soy sauce 1 t. basil, dried
2	In another sauté pan add oil and cook chicken until done, about 8 minutes. Add to the pot with the water and barley cover and simmer 30 minutes, stirring occasionally.	1 T. olive oil 4 chicken breast, boneless, skinless 8 C. filtered water ¾ C. barley
3	Dice the cauliflower into bite size pieces and add to soup and cook another 15 minutes	1 small cauliflower, diced
4	Reduce heat and add peas and lemon juice and simmer until just hot.	10 oz. frozen peas 2-3 t. lemon juice
5	Adjust seasonings to taste and serve.	¼ t. sea salt ¼ t. pepper

Chicken and Spinach Soup with Fresh Pesto

(1 ½ cup serving: 264, 18 g protein, 8 g fat, 30 g carbohydrates)

Serves 6-8

1	Heat the oil in a large Dutch oven over medium heat. Add the carrots and the chicken; cook turning the chicken and stirring frequently about 3-4 minutes.	2 t. olive oil ½ carrot, chopped 2-3 chicken breast, boned and skinned
2	Add garlic and cook 1 minute, stirring. Add broth and marjoram bring to a boil and then reduce to a simmer for 5 minutes.	1 clove of garlic, minced 5 C. chicken broth 1½ t. marjoram, dried
3	With a slotted spoon take the chicken pieces out and dice; set aside.	
4	Add spinach and beans to the soup and bring to a low boil for 5 minutes.	14 oz. baby spinach leaves 1 15-oz. can great northern beans, rinsed
5	In a food processor combine oil, mozzarella cheese, and basil. Process until course paste forms adding water if necessary.	1 T. olive oil ¼ C. mozzarella cheese, grated ½ C. basil leaves, fresh
6	Stir chicken into soup along with the cheese pesto. Season with pepper. Heat until hot and serve.	¼ t. pepper

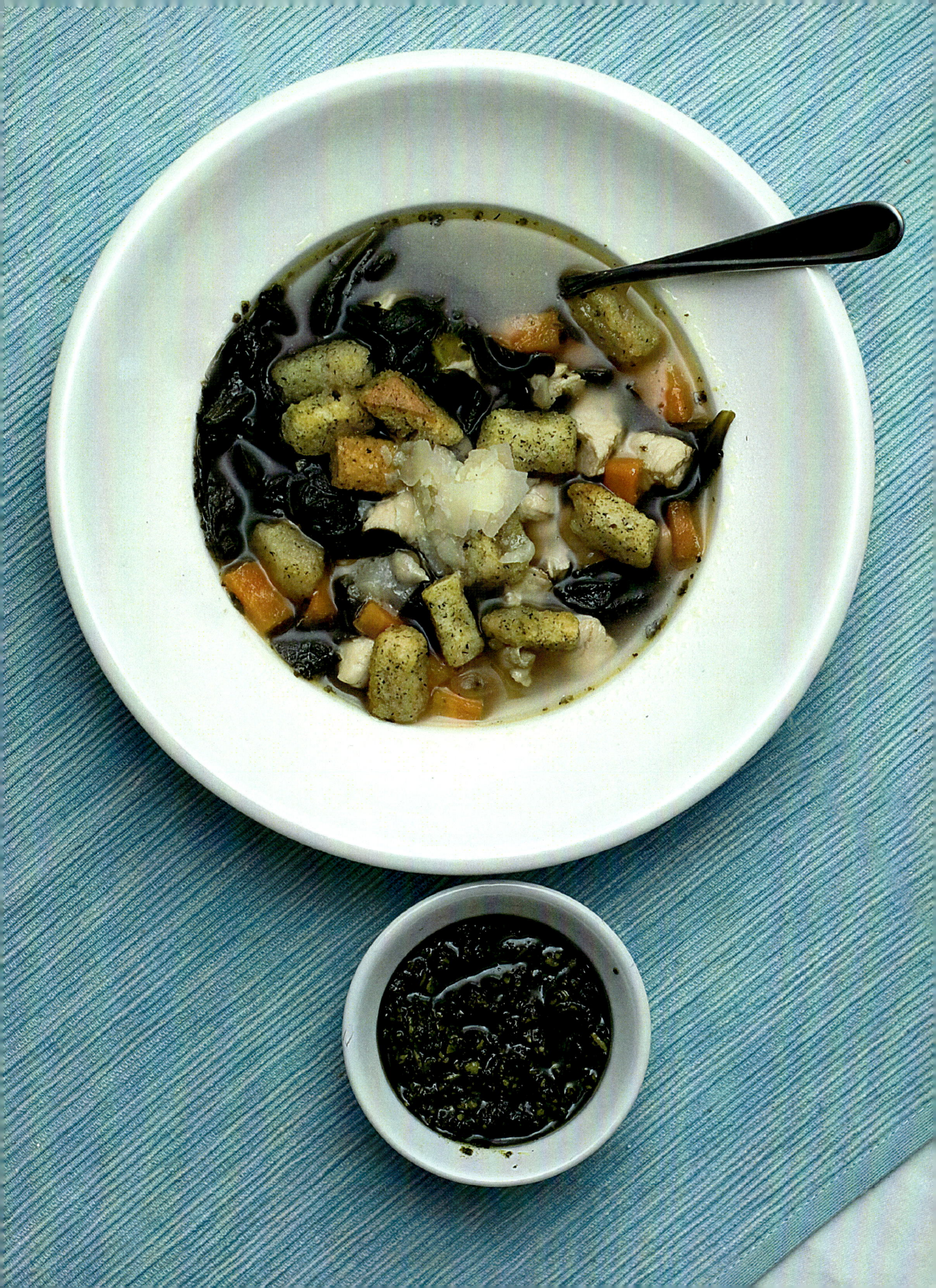

Coconut Curry Noodle Soup
(Calories: 195, 14 g protein, 6 g fat, 20 g carbohydrates)

Serves 4-6

1	Steam the spinach and snow peas; 2 minutes.	3 C. spinach leaves ¾ lb. snow peas
2	Cook noodles in water about 8 minutes. Strain; set aside.	¾ lb. Soba (buckwheat) noodles 1 qt. filtered water
3	Transfer the spinach, snow peas and noodles into bowls.	
4	Meanwhile in a large saucepan, heat oil and sauté scallions for 4 minutes; set aside.	1 T. coconut oil 3 scallions, thinly sliced
5	In a pan sauté the garlic, curry paste, curry powder, coriander and turmeric for 30 seconds. Add the stock and bring to a boil cooking about 3 minutes.	2 cloves garlic, minced 2 t. curry paste 1 ½ t. curry powder ½ t. coriander ½ t. turmeric 6 C. chicken broth
6	Add the coconut milk, fish sauce and maple syrup and bring to a boil and simmer for 5 minutes.	1 can coconut milk 2 T. fish sauce 1 T. maple syrup
7	Add the chicken, parsley and heat through; season with sea salt. Ladle soup over the noodles and serve with cooked scallions and lime wedges.	1-2 C. cooked chicken breast, shredded ¼ C. parsley leaves ¼ t. sea salt Lime wedges

Split Pea with Ham Soup

(Calories: 328, 28 g protein, 4 g fat, 45 g carbohydrates)

Serves 6-8

1	In a large soup pot heat oil and add onion, celery, apple and parsley. Reduce heat and add spices sautéing and stirring often until vegetables are done about 10 minutes.	1-2 T. olive oil 1 large onion, chopped 2 stalks celery, trimmed and chopped 1 green apple, chopped ¼ C. parsley leaves, chopped 1 T. curry powder 2 t. ground cumin 2 t. whole mustard seeds 1 t. coriander 1 t. ground turmeric
2	Stir in split peas and water to cover them by two inches. Bring to a boil and then reduce heat and cover; simmer one hour or whenever the peas are soft and ready to puree.	1½ C. split peas, rinsed 1½ qts. filtered water
3	Puree in blender or in a food processor. Return to pot.	
4	On low heat stir in lemon juice and ham. Season with salt and pepper.	1 T. lemon juice 8-16 oz. cooked ham, diced ¼ t. sea salt ¼ t. pepper
5	Serve hot. May be refrigerated 2-3 days.	

Split Pea with Spiced Yogurt
(1Cup Calories: 250, 20 g protein, 3 g fat, 37 g carbohydrate)

Serves 4-8

1	Heat butter and oil in a pan and add onion, garlic, ginger, bay leaf and salt.	1 T. organic butter 1 T. olive oil 1 large onion, minced 2 cloves garlic, minced 1 1" piece ginger root, peeled and minced 1 bay leaf ½ t. sea salt
2	Add cumin and cloves and cook 3 minute.	1 t. cumin 3 cloves, powdered
3	Rinse and drain the peas and add to onion mixture.	1 2/3 C. split peas
4	Dice the celery and add along with the filtered water and bring to a boil; lower heat and simmer 1 hour. Return to pot and add ham.	2 stalks celery 7 C. filtered water 16 oz. cooked ham, diced
5	To make Spiced Yogurt: Blend together yogurt and spices.	½ C. plain yogurt ½ t. turmeric ½ t. paprika ¼ t. cayenne ¼ t. cumin
6	Place soup in bowls and top with yogurt.	

Cauliflower Cheese Soup
(Calories: 218, 7 g protein, 10 g fat, 25 g carbohydrates)

Serves 4-6

1	Core cauliflower and cut into florets-reserve 6-8 for garnish.	1 large cauliflower
2	In a large pan heat butter and oil and sauté garlic and onion until softened. Add cauliflower and chicken broth and bring to a boil; reduce and simmer for 20-25 minutes.	1 T. butter 1 T. olive oil 2 cloves garlic, minced 3 C. onion, chopped 4 C. chicken broth
3	Puree mixture in blender and return to pan.	
4	On low heat slowly add milk, cayenne, nutmeg and chives, stirring constantly until the soup is hot.	1 C. whole milk ¼ t. cayenne pepper ½ t. nutmeg, ground 3 T. chives, chopped
5	Cut cheese into small chunks and add to soup stirring until melted.	4 oz. goat feta cheese, cubed
6	Add salt and pepper.	¼ t. sea salt ¼ t. pepper
7	While soup is heating, sauté reserved cauliflower florets in oil. Roll florets in cornmeal and garlic salt and drop into soup. Sprinkle with chives and paprika.	1 T. olive oil 1 T. cornmeal ½ t. garlic salt ½ t. paprika 1 T. chopped chives

Black Bean Chili
(Calories: 350, 18 g protein, 4 g fat, 28 g carbohydrates)

Serves 8-10

1	Pick over the beans and discard any broken beans or rocks. Soak over night in enough filtered water to cover by 2 inches.	3 C. organic dried black beans (may use 3 cans)
2	Drain the beans and place in a large soup pot and add water to cover beans, approximately 1 quart. Bring to a boil, reduce heat, cover and simmer for one hour. Add water if necessary. If using canned beans heat in a large soup pot over medium to low heat.	1 qt. filtered water
3	In a pan heat oil and sauté onions, celery, carrots and garlic until light brown about 8 minutes.	2 t. olive oil 1 large onion, chopped 2-3 stalks celery, chopped 2-3 carrots, chopped 2-3 cloves garlic. minced
4	Deglaze the pan using tequila or lime juice scraping up any brown bits.	1 T. tequila (may use lime juice)
5	Stir in spices and chipotle peppers with adobo sauce. Add ground meat and cook until meat is brown about 5 minutes	1 t. oregano, dried ½ t. cumin ½ t. coriander 2 chipotle peppers seeded and chopped in adobo sauce* or 1 T. cayenne pepper 1 lb. ground turkey breast

6	Add the onion mixture to the bean pot. Add broth and bring to a boil, lower, cover and simmer for 1 hour.	1-2 C. chicken broth
7	Add sea salt, lime juice just before serving.	½ t. sea salt juice of one lime
8	May freeze for up to 3 months.	

Tip: *Chipotle peppers in adobo sauce are not option purple, but it is such a small percentage of the meal it will be fine. You may exclude them and use cayenne pepper for flavor instead.

61

Green Beans with Pecans Pg 68

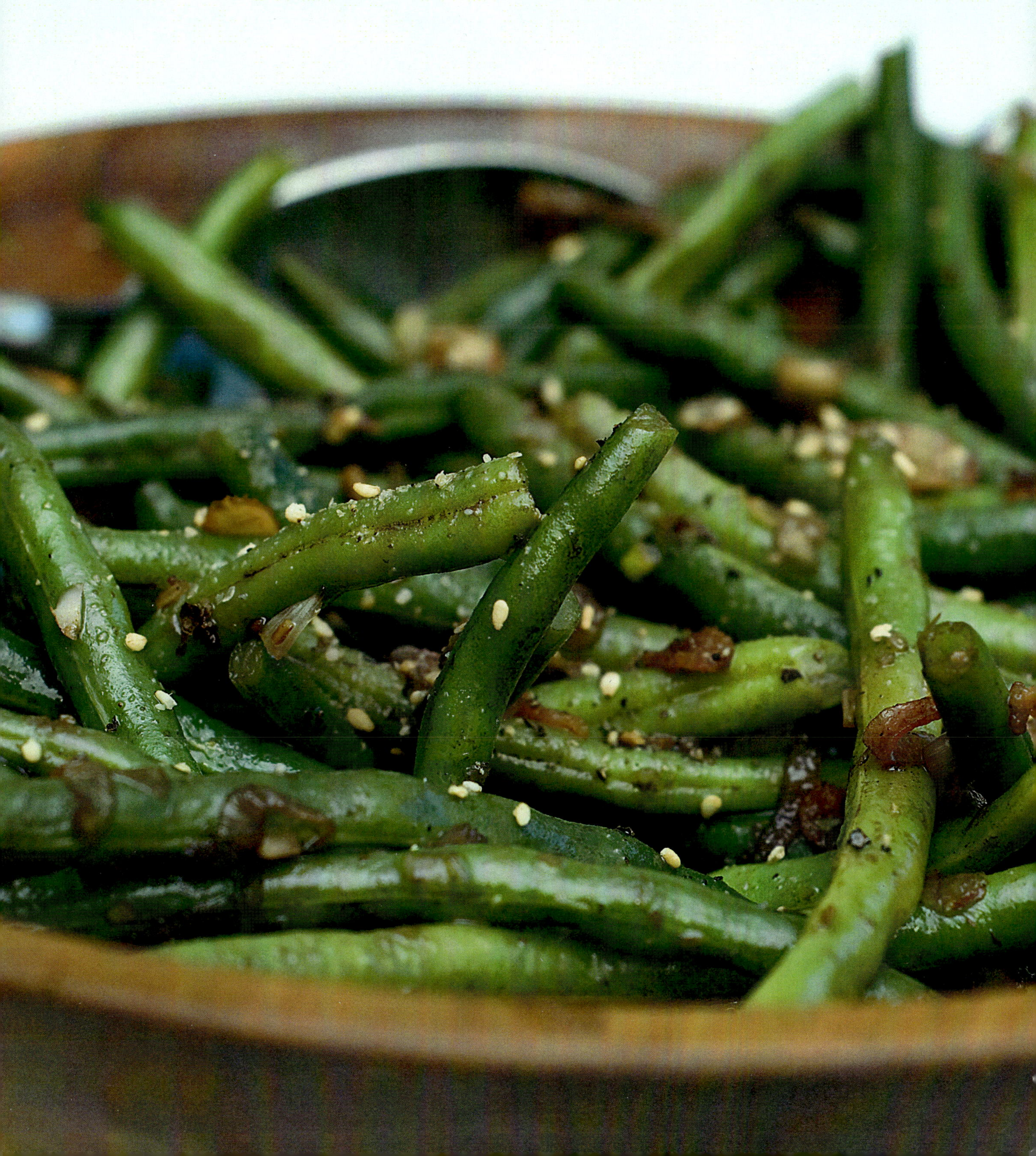

Vegetables and more

45% of your diet should come from carbohydrates.

Sautéed Vegetables

(1 cup: Calories: 100, 4 g protein, 5 g fat, 15 g carbohydrates)

Serves 4-6

1	Heat oil in large skillet over medium heat and add onions; sauté 5 minutes	1-2 T. olive oil or coconut oil 2 onions, sliced
2	Add mushrooms and cook 3 minutes.	6 oz. mushrooms, sliced
3	Add vegetables and salt and pepper and sauté another 4-5 minutes. Extras can be refrigerated for 3-4 days.	½ lb. asparagus, chopped ½ lb. green beans, chopped

Tip: You can use any vegetable from your diet. Serve with Almond Crusted Chicken and a green salad.

Sautéed Vegetables

(1 cup: Calories: 100, 4 g protein, 5 g fat, 15 g carbohydrates)

Serves 4-6

1	Heat oil in large skillet over medium heat and add shallots ; sauté 5 minutes	1-2 T. olive oil or coconut oil 2 shallots, sliced
2	Add broccoli and cook 3 minutes.	8 oz. broccoli, sliced
3	Add vegetables and salt and pepper and sauté another 4-5 minutes. Extras can be refrigerated for 3-4 days.	½ lb. zucchini, chopped ½ lb. red peppers, chopped

Tip: You can use any vegetable from your diet. Serve with Almond Crusted Chicken and a green salad.

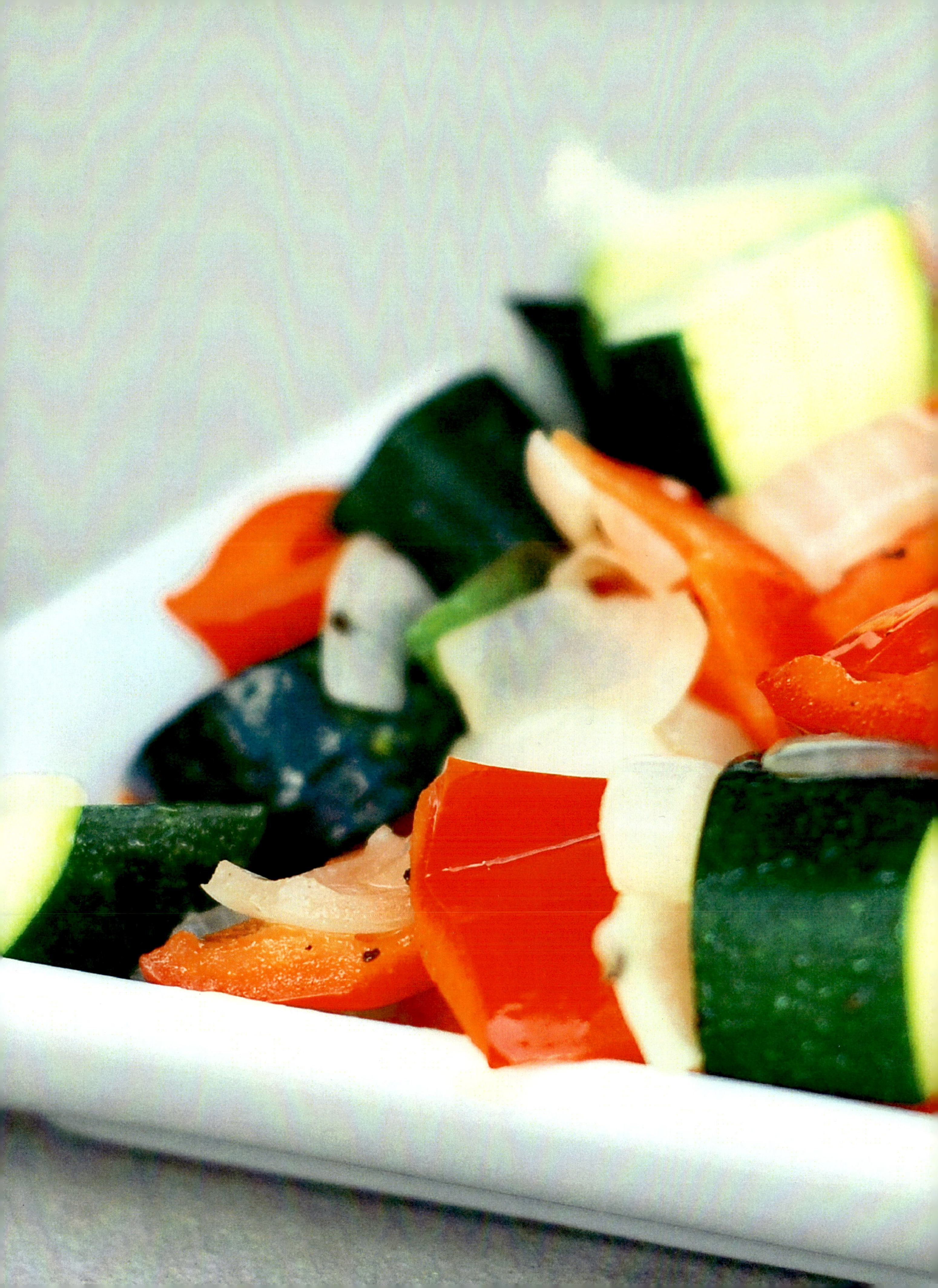

Cheese and Spinach Stuffed Portobello
(Calories: 201, 14 g protein, 10 g fat, 13 g carbohydrates)

Serves 4

1	Preheat oven to 450° F	
2	Coat a rimmed baking sheet with oil and place the mushrooms gill side up, sprinkled with salt and pepper. Roast for 20-25 minutes.	4 large Portobello mushrooms ¼ t. sea salt ¼ t. pepper
3	Mash ricotta, spinach, mozzarella, olives, Italian seasoning and black pepper in a medium bowl.	1 C. ricotta cheese 1 C. fresh spinach leaves finely chopped ¼ C. mozzarella cheese 2 T. Kalamata olives, finely chopped ½ t. Italian seasoning ¼ t. black pepper
4	Warm the marinara sauce on the stove until hot.	¾ C. prepared marinara sauce
5	When mushrooms are tender, carefully pour out any liquid accumulated in the caps. Return to baking sheet gill side up. Spread 1 tablespoon of marinara sauce over each cap; mound a generous 1/3 cup ricotta filling into each of the caps and sprinkle with the cheese.	¼ C. mozzarella cheese
6	Bake until hot, about 10 minutes. Serve with the remaining marinara sauce.	

Prosciutto Wrapped Broccoli
(Calories: 39, 3 g protein, 2 g fat, 3 g carbohydrates)

Serves 4

1	Preheat grill to medium	
2	Toss broccoli with oil, salt and pepper in a medium bowl.	16 broccoli florets, cleaned and trimmed 1 t. olive oil ½ t. sea salt ¼ t. pepper
3	Wrap 1 length of prosciutto around the middle of 4 asparagus spears.	2 very thin slices prosciutto cut in half lengthwise
4	Grill the broccoli in bundles on low turning once or twice until done about 10 minutes. Serve immediately.	

Tip: This makes a great appetizer.

1. Restaurant Green Beans
2. Green Beans with Pecans
3 .Green Bean Pate with Basil

1	Take fresh green beans, a large pot of water and 2 T. salt. (The salt sets the color and you rinse it off with cold water). Bring salted water to a rolling boil, put in green beans and cook 6-8 minutes. Rinse and drain on paper towel. Use in salads or add butter and serve.	1 lb. fresh green beans cleaned and trimmed. 1 qt. water 1 T. sea salt
2	Cook beans until tender about 6 minutes. Meanwhile, heat oil and butter in a pan and sauté scallions until softened. Stir in parsley and savory. Add the beans and almonds, season with salt and pepper and serve.	1½ lb. green beans cleaned and trimmed 2 T. organic butter 1 T. olive oil ¼ C. scallions, chopped ¼ C. fresh parsley, chopped ½ t. savory, dried 1 C. almonds, sliced ¼ t. sea salt ¼ t. pepper
3	Steam the beans about 6 minutes. In skillet heat oil; add onion and sauté until soft. Cool. In a food processor, process the beans, onion, eggs, basil and lemon rind until roughly pureed. Remove from bowl and mix in just enough mayonnaise. Stir in salt and pepper to taste. Chill.	½ lb. fresh green beans, cleaned and trimmed 1 T. olive oil 1 onion, chopped 3 hard boiled eggs 1 t. lemon rind 3 T. fresh basil, chopped 1-2 T. mayonnaise ¼ t. sea salt ¼ t. pepper

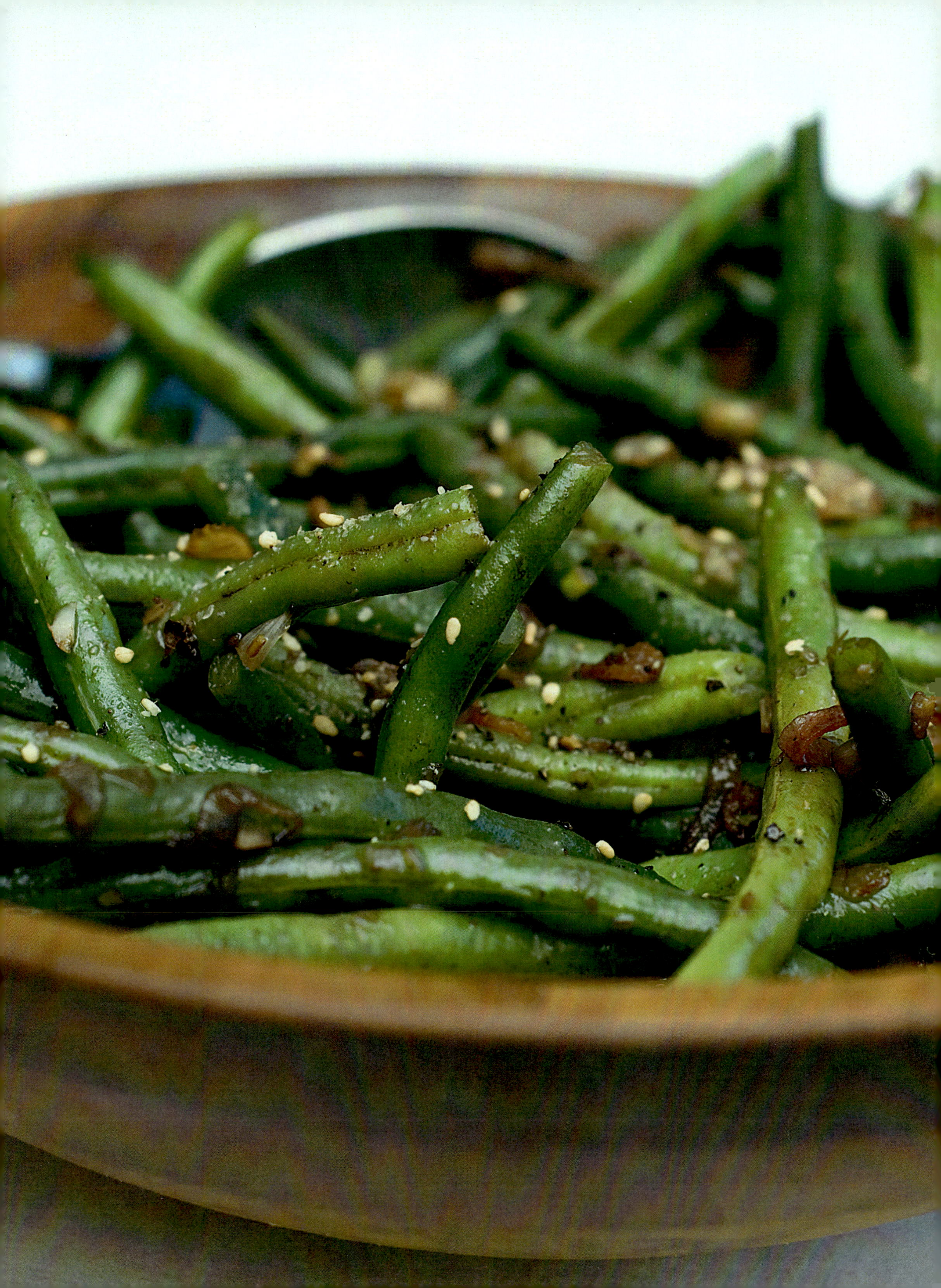

Brussels Sprouts with Bacon-Balsamic Vinaigrette
(Calories: 164, 2 g protein, 4 g fat, 30 g carbohydrates)

Serves 6-8

1	Steam sprouts for 8 minutes; drain and cut in half and rinse with cold water.	2 lb. Brussels sprouts, trimmed
2	Cook bacon in a small skillet over medium heat until crisp. Remove and crumble; set a side.	2 slices bacon
3	Add shallots to bacon pan and sauté for 1 minute. Add walnuts and sauté another minute. Remove form pan and cool.	¼ C. shallots, minced 3 T. chopped walnuts, toasted
4	In a bowl add vinegar and maple syrup and stir until dissolved. Add walnuts and shallots and mix together. Divide Brussels sprouts into 6 plates pour vinaigrette over them and then add crumbled bacon and serve warm or cold.	¼ balsamic vinegar 1 t. maple syrup

Tip: This dish can be served with one of my beef dishes to make a balanced meal.

Green Beans with Mushrooms

(Calories: 138, 2 g protein, 10 g fat, 10 g carbohydrates)

Serves 4

#		
1	Brown the onions in the butter and add mushrooms; cook 2 minutes.	2 T. raw butter ½ onion, diced ½ lb. mushrooms, sliced
2	Clean and blanche the green beans in salted water for 30 seconds. Drain.	1 lb. green beans cut into 2 inch lengths
3	Add the chicken broth to the mushrooms and onions and bring to a boil. Add paprika, dill and salt and pepper to taste. Boil for 5 minutes.	1 C. chicken broth ¼ t. paprika ¼ t. dill, dried ¼ t. sea salt ¼ t. pepper
4	Add the green beans and sour cream. Simmer on low for 8-10 minutes and serve.	½ C. sour cream

Blue Cheese-Walnut Broccoli
(Calories: 163, 6 g protein, 12 g fat, 10g carbohydrates)

Serves 4

1	Clean, trim and cut the florets. Steam for 6-8 minutes. Transfer to a bowl and add olive oil, salt and pepper and toss.	1 lb. broccoli florets 1 T. olive oil ¼ t. sea salt ¼ t. pepper
2	Toast the walnuts until light brown but not burnt about 2 minutes.	1/3 C. walnuts, chopped
3	Toss the broccoli with blue cheese and divide into four plates and sprinkle each serving with the walnuts.	1/3 C. blue cheese, crumbled

Tip: This is a great side dish served with a protein such as Bison Steaks or Pear Cranberry Stuffed Pork Roast.

Stuffed Butternut Squash
(Calories: 300, 18 g protein, 8 g fat, 39 g carbohydrates)

Serves 6-8

1	Preheat oven to 375° F	
2	Trim the ends off the squash, cut in half and scoop out ½ the flesh and cube it; keeping it for the stuffing but leaving about ¼ inch shell. Sprinkle inside with soy sauce and lemon juice. Bake skin side up for 35 minutes. .	2 small butternut squash 1 T. tamari wheat free soy sauce 1 T. lemon juice
3	Let cooked squash cool.	
4	Meanwhile make the stuffing: In a large skillet heat oil and cook the turkey or beef until done. To the skillet add the vegetables and spices in the order listed. Stir in the squash scooped out along with the meat; simmer about ten minutes.	1 T. olive oil 1 lb. ground turkey or beef 1½ C. celery, diced ½ C. shallots, diced 1 C. red pepper, chopped 1½ C. tomatoes, seeded and chopped ½ C. sunflower seeds, lightly toasted ¼ C. raisins (optional) 2 t. cumin 1 t. coriander pinch of sage ¼ t. sea salt ¼ t. pepper
5	Stuff the squash shells; top with breadcrumbs and cheese. Place in a shallow pan. Pour water in pan; bake for 45 min. Cut in serving sizes and serve.	¼ C. bread crumbs ¼ C. parmesan cheese ¼ C. water

Mushroom and Spinach Stuffed Summer Squash
(Calories: 300, 10 g protein, 18 g fat, 25 g carbohydrates)

Serves 6-8

1	Preheat oven to 350° F	
2	Slice the squash in half and scoop out the flesh making a boat. Set aside	4 medium squash or 8 small (any variety summer squash)
3	In a skillet sauté in butter and oil the onions, garlic until soft.	1 T. butter 1 T. olive oil 1 onion, minced 2 garlic cloves, minced
4	Add mushrooms, sherry, dill, and soy sauce and cook for 5 minutes. When the mushrooms are tender, remove from heat and set a side.	3 C. portabello mushrooms, chopped 1 T. dry sherry 1 t. dill, dried 2 t. tamari wheat free soy sauce
5	While the mushrooms are cooking, rinse and steam the spinach until wilted about 5 minutes; drain and add to mushroom mixture. Stir in quinoa and salt and pepper.	5 oz. spinach leaves 1 C. quinoa, cooked ¼ t. sea salt ¼ t. pepper
6	Pour the water in the bottom of an 8x10 inch pan. Press and mound the filing into the squash boats. Sprinkle cheese on top and bake for 30 minutes covered with foil. Uncover and bake 10 minutes more. Serve immediately.	½ C. water ½ C. grated mozzarella cheese

Mediterranean Vegetable Quinoa
(Calories: 220, 4 g protein, 3 g fat, 47 g carbohydrates)

Serves 6-8

1	Heat oil in large skillet. Add onion, garlic and cook until brown about 5 minutes.	1 T. olive oil 1 onion, chopped 2-3 cloves garlic, minced
2	Add vegetables and spices and cook for 5- 8 minutes.	1 fennel bulb, chopped 2 carrot, chopped 1 C. summer squash, chopped ½ C. celery, chopped ¼ C. oil-cured olives, chopped 1 ½ t. basil, dried 1½ t. oregano, dried 1 t. sea salt ¼ t. cinnamon
3	Thoroughly rinse quinoa and then put into the boiling water or broth, lower heat and simmer 20 minutes. Drain off any extra water from the quinoa.	1½ C. quinoa 2½ C. water or chicken broth
4	Add quinoa to vegetables and stir in lemon juice cooking for 5 more minutes. Add fresh herbs and serve. May be refrigerated 4 days.	1-3 T. lemon juice ¼ C. fresh parsley or basil

Tip: To make this into complete meal combine with Chicken Crusted in Almonds.

Mashed Cauliflower "Potatoes"
(Calories: 160, 4 g protein, 7 g fat, 20 g carbohydrates)

Serves 4-6

1	Steam the cauliflower until soft 6-8 minutes.	4 C. cauliflower florets
2	Puree in a food processor or mash them like you would potatoes.	
3	Add butter and cream. Season with salt and pepper. Serve immediately.	2 T. butter ¼ C. half and half or raw cream ¼ t. sea salt ¼ t. pepper

Tip: These can replace mashed potatoes easily. With a Glycemic Index of "0" compared with mashed potatoes at "73" it makes a great choice.

Twice Baked Potatoes
(Calories: 290, 5 g protein, 14 g fat, 30 g carbohydrates)

Serves 6-8

1	Preheat oven to 425° F	
2	Wash and dry potatoes; rub with olive oil and fork each one. Place in oven for one hour.	4 medium russet potatoes 1 T. olive oil
3	Cut the potato in half and scoop out the inside and place half the flesh in a bowl.	
4	In the bowl add milk; whipping the mixture until all the lumps are out. Add the shallots and the steamed vegetables for 6 minutes. Add salt and pepper; mixing well.	½ C. whole milk 2 T. raw butter 2-4 shallots, minced ¼ C. broccoli, diced ¼ C. red pepper, diced ¼ C. zucchini, diced ¼ t. sea salt ¼ t. pepper
5	Put mixture back into the potato skins. Sprinkle with cheese. Bake at 350° F for 15 minutes. Serve immediately.	½ C. Swiss cheese, grated

Tip: Serve with any of the beef recipes. Can be made ahead of time and baked before serving.

Enchiladas Pg 100

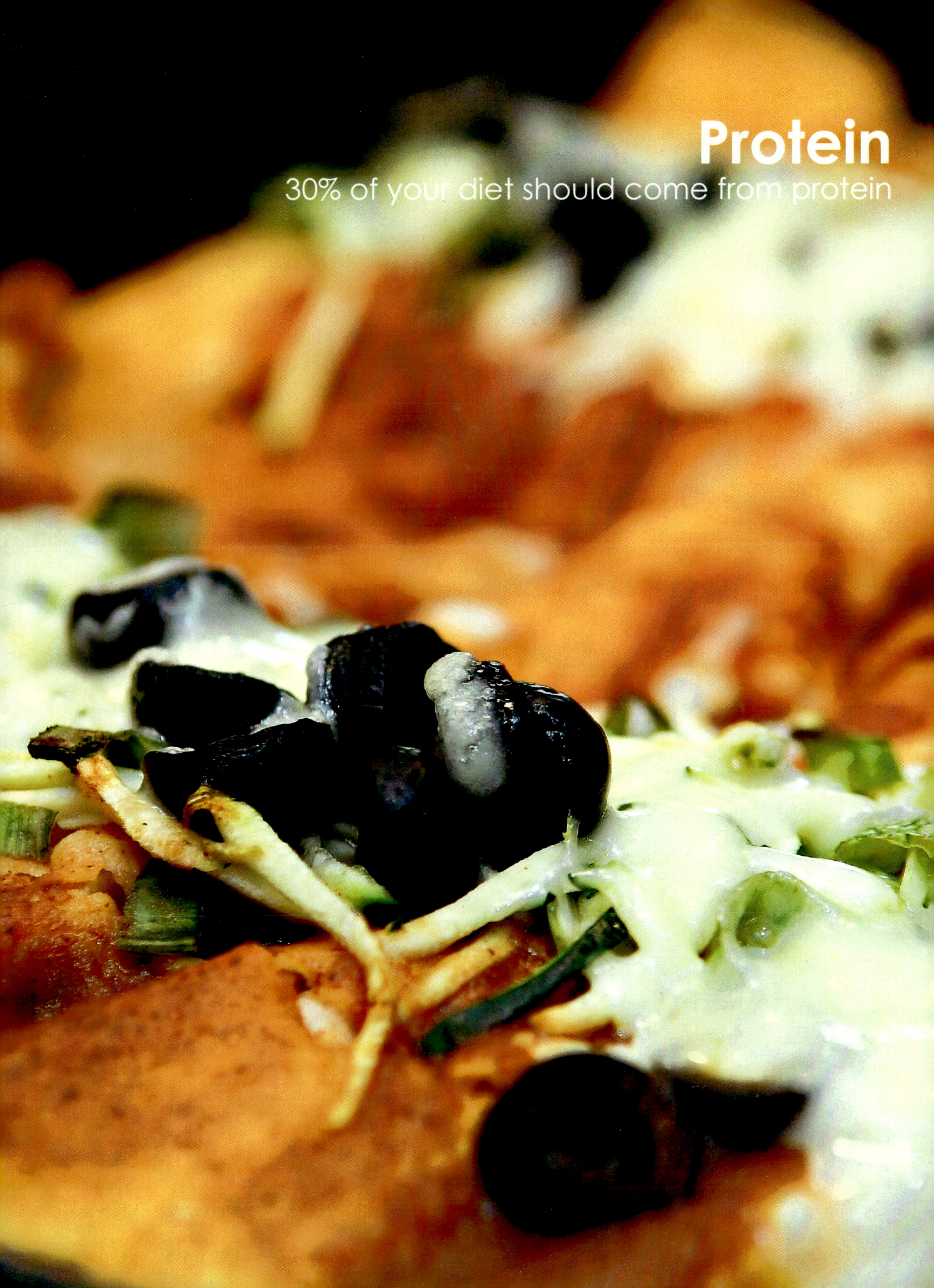
Protein
30% of your diet should come from protein

Chicken Curry

(Calories: 350, 27 g protein (with chicken), 14 g fat, 29 g carbohydrates)

Serves 4-6

1	Sauté onions in ghee or butter.	3 T. ghee or unsalted butter 1 C. onion, chopped
2	Add spices and stir for 3 minutes.	1 T. fenugreek seeds, ground ¼ t. cayenne pepper 1 t. coriander, ground 2 T. turmeric 1 t. cumin, ground ½ t. cloves, ground 1 t. cardamom, ground
3	Add chicken stock and lemon juice and bring to a boil.	2-3 C. chicken stock 1-2 lemons, juiced
4	Stir in the garlic, coconut milk and cream. Simmer uncovered about 15 minutes, stirring frequently until sauce is reduced and thickened.	1 C. crème fraiche 1 can coconut milk 2 garlic cloves, minced
5	Serve over chicken with green onions and condiments on a bed of Quinoa.	4-6 chicken breast boneless, skinless, cooked 2-3 green onions, chopped 2 C. Quinoa, cooked

Tip: Serve with Fresh Fig Salad.

Chicken with Capers
(Calories: 160, 27 g protein, 5 g fat, 12 g carbohydrates)

Serves 4

1	Sprinkle salt and pepper over chicken.	8 chicken thighs ¼ t. sea salt ¼ t. pepper
2	Heat oil in skillet over medium heat. Add chicken and sauté 6 minutes each side or until done. Remove and set aside keeping warm.	1 T. olive oil
3	To skillet add broth, salt and pepper lemon juice and capers. Stir scraping skillet to loosen brown bits. Cook liquid until reduced to ¼ cup (about 2 minutes).	½ C. chicken broth ¼ t. sea salt ¼ t. pepper 2 T. lemon juice 3 T. capers, rinsed
4	Stir in the parsley and spoon over the chicken and serve.	¼ C. parsley, chopped

Tip: This dish needs to be served with the appropriate option vegetable such as Prosciutto wrapped Broccoli to balance the meal.

Chicken Crusted in Almonds
(Calories: 150, 28 g protein, 5 g fat, 3 g carbohydrates)

Serves 6-8

1	Cut chicken in half and place between two sheets of plastic and pound until ¼ inch thick or twice the original size.	6-8 boneless, skinless chicken breasts
2	Mix together the almond meal, garlic, lemon zest and salt and pepper and place in a pie tin.	½ C. almond meal 1-2 cloves garlic, minced zest of one organic lemon ¼ t. sea salt ¼ t. pepper
3	In another pie tin crack an egg and whip with a small amount of water until frothy.	1 egg ¼ C. water
4	Heat oil in a large skillet over medium flame and place the chicken dredged in egg and then almond mixture into it. Sauté each side 2-4 minutes until light brown. Serve immediately. Extras can be refrigerated for 2-3 days.	2 T. olive oil or coconut oil

Tip: This dish goes perfect with Sautéed Vegetable and a green salad. You can also use this crust to pan fry halibut.

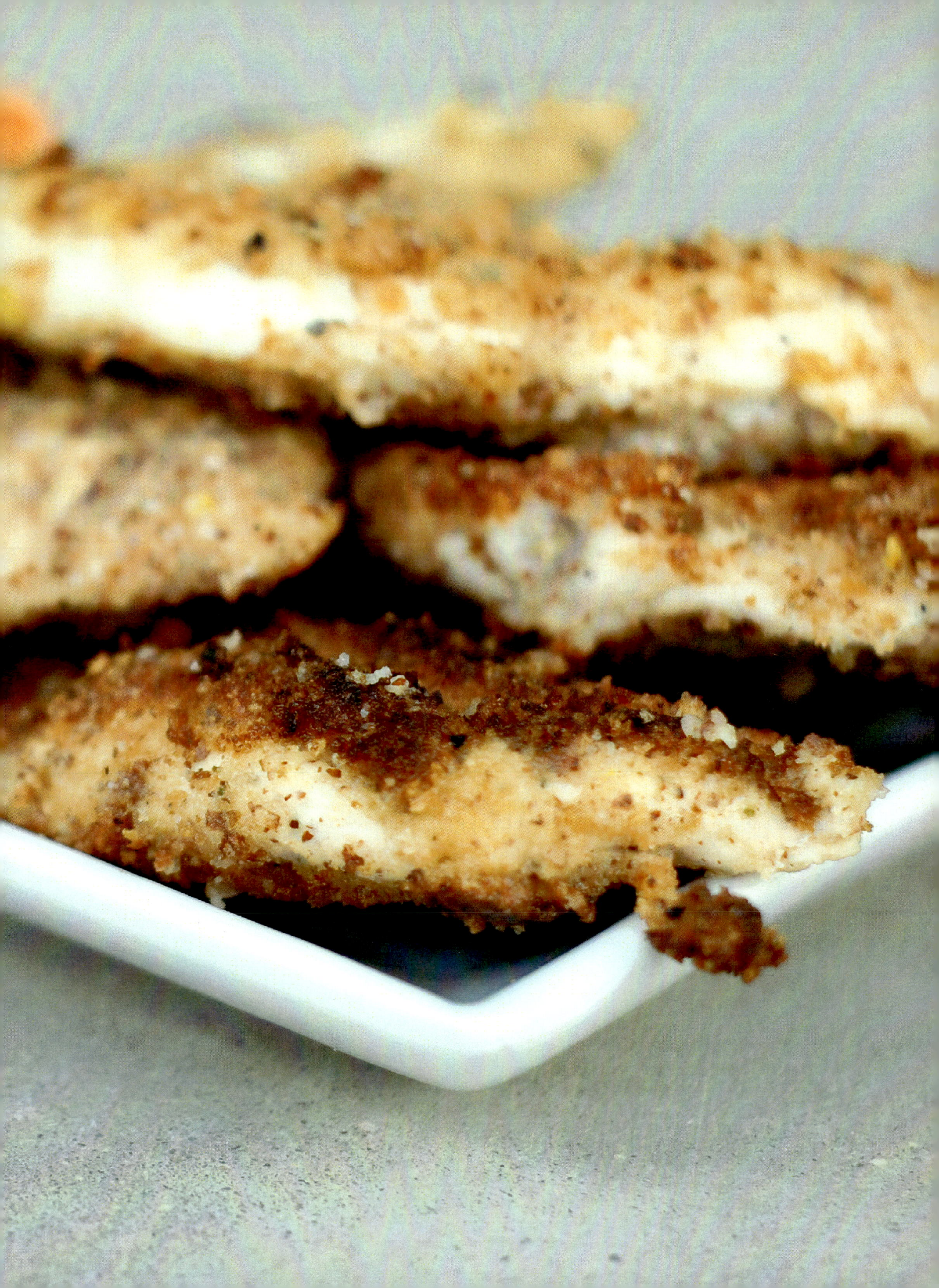

Orange-Ginger Chicken
(Calories: 245, 27 g protein, 4 g fat, 25 g carbohydrates)

Serves 4

1	Heat oil in a large skillet over medium heat. Add chicken and sauté for 5-6 minutes each side.	4 chicken breast, boned and skinned ½ t. dark sesame oil ½ t. chili oil
2	Add marmalade and other ingredients and cook for 2 minutes or until bubbly.	1/3 C. orange marmalade 3 T. soy sauce 1 T. ginger, minced 1 T. water 2 cloves garlic, minced
3	Serve immediately.	

Tip: Serve this with Cauliflower Brie soup. Remember this can be a green choice if you use thighs, but you must change the vegetable choice.

Slow/Low Heat Cooking Techniques

1	Preheat oven to 225° F	Bake 5 minutes per oz. of food
2	Using a glass roasting dish with lid, place chicken skin side up on the bottom. Place lid on securely; Bake for 1 hour and 20 minutes.	1 lb. chicken thighs, breasts or legs
3	Combine ingredients and make into four patties; place in a glass dish and put lid on; bake 1 hour and 20 minutes.	1 lb. of ground beef, turkey or bison ¼- ½ t. herbs (your choice) ¼ t. sea salt ¼ t. pepper
4	Place in a glass dish, drizzle with butter or olive oil, salt and pepper and bake covered for 1 hour and 20 minutes.	1 lb. of any firm fish (salmon, halibut, cod bass) 1 T. olive oil or butter ¼ t. sea salt ¼ t. pepper

Tip: Use this technique for vegetables as well. Place squash (whole) pierce the skin and bake 5 minutes per ounce in a glass dish with lid on.

Rolled Chicken Stuffed with Vegetables
(Calories: 250, 24 g protein, 10 g fat, 16 g carbohydrates)

Serves 4

1	In a small sauté pan place balsamic vinegar on medium heat and heat until liquid is reduce ½ the original amount making a reduction. Set aside.	½ C. balsamic vinegar (optional)
2	Pound the chicken between two sheets of plastic until ¼ inch thick.	8 chicken thighs
3	Steam the broccoli florets 5 minutes and remove from steamer, pat dry.	8 oz. of broccoli
4	Add water to egg and beat until frothy and place in a pie tin. In another pie tin place almond meal, salt and pepper.	1 egg 1/8 C. water ¼ t. sea salt ¼ t. pepper ½ C. bread crumbs
5	Place ¼ of the broccoli on each chicken piece along with the slice of Swiss cheese and roll up and secure with pick.	4 oz. Swiss cheese, sliced
6	Dip rolled chicken into egg mixture and then into almond meal. Sauté in oil for 10-15 minutes until light brown and done. Serve drizzled with balsamic.	

Rolled Chicken Stuffed with Vegetables
(Calories: 250, 24 g protein, 10 g fat, 16 g carbohydrates)

Serves 4

1	In a small sauté pan place balsamic vinegar on medium heat and heat until liquid is reduce ½ the original amount making a reduction. Set aside.	½ C. balsamic vinegar (optional)
2	Pound the chicken between two sheets of plastic until ¼ inch thick.	4 boneless, skinless breast
3	Steam the spinach and drain all water off. If using broccoli; steam florets 5 minutes and remove from steamer, pat dry.	8 oz. of spinach
4	Add water to egg and beat until frothy and place in a pie tin. In another pie tin place almond meal, salt and pepper.	1 egg 1/8 C. water ¼ t. sea salt ¼ t. pepper ½ C. almond meal
5	Place ¼ of the spinach or 1 floret of broccoli on each chicken piece along with feta cheese and roll up and secure with pick.	4 oz. goat feta cheese
6	Dip rolled chicken into egg mixture and then into almond meal. Sauté in oil for 10-15 minutes until light brown and done. Serve drizzled with balsamic.	

Salmon Cakes
(Calories: 150, 17 g protein, 7 g fat, 8 g carbohydrates)

Serves 4

1	In a food processor process ingredients until minced fine.	½ C. red and green pepper, minced 1 C. bread crumbs 1/3 C. cilantro ¼ C. shallot, minced 1 egg 1 T. lemon juice 1 T. Tabasco sauce ¼ t. sea salt ¼ t. pepper
2	Combine the salmon with the mixture and form into patties on waxed paper and chill for 30 minutes.	1 lb. cooked salmon, diced
3	Heat oil in skillet over medium heat. Cook the patties about 2-3 minutes per side. Transfer to oven and cook through about 4 minutes. Serve immediately.	1-2 T. olive oil or coconut oil

Tip: This served on a bed of lettuce with sliced tomato makes a complete meal.

Shrimp Jambalaya
(Calories: 350, 22 g protein, 12 g fat, 38 g carbohydrates)

Serves 8-10

1	Brown the sausage in oil and sauté over medium heat about 3 minutes.	2 T. olive oil 5-6 turkey, chicken or pork sausages
2	Stir in shallots and peppers sauté 5 minutes.	1½ C. shallots, chopped 1 C. red bell pepper, chopped 1 C. green bell pepper, chopped
3	Add shrimp and cook 3 minutes stirring constantly.	1 lb. shrimp, peeled, deveined
4	Stir in tomatoes and cooked rice for 3-4 minutes heating through.	4 C. tomatoes, chopped 3 C. rice, cooked
5	Season with Tabasco sauce and salt and pepper.	2 t. Tabasco sauce ¼ t. sea salt ¼ t. pepper
6	Garnish with shallots and serve.	¼ C. shallots, chopped fine

Tip: Serve with steamed broccoli or Brussels sprouts with Bacon-Balsamic Vinaigrette.

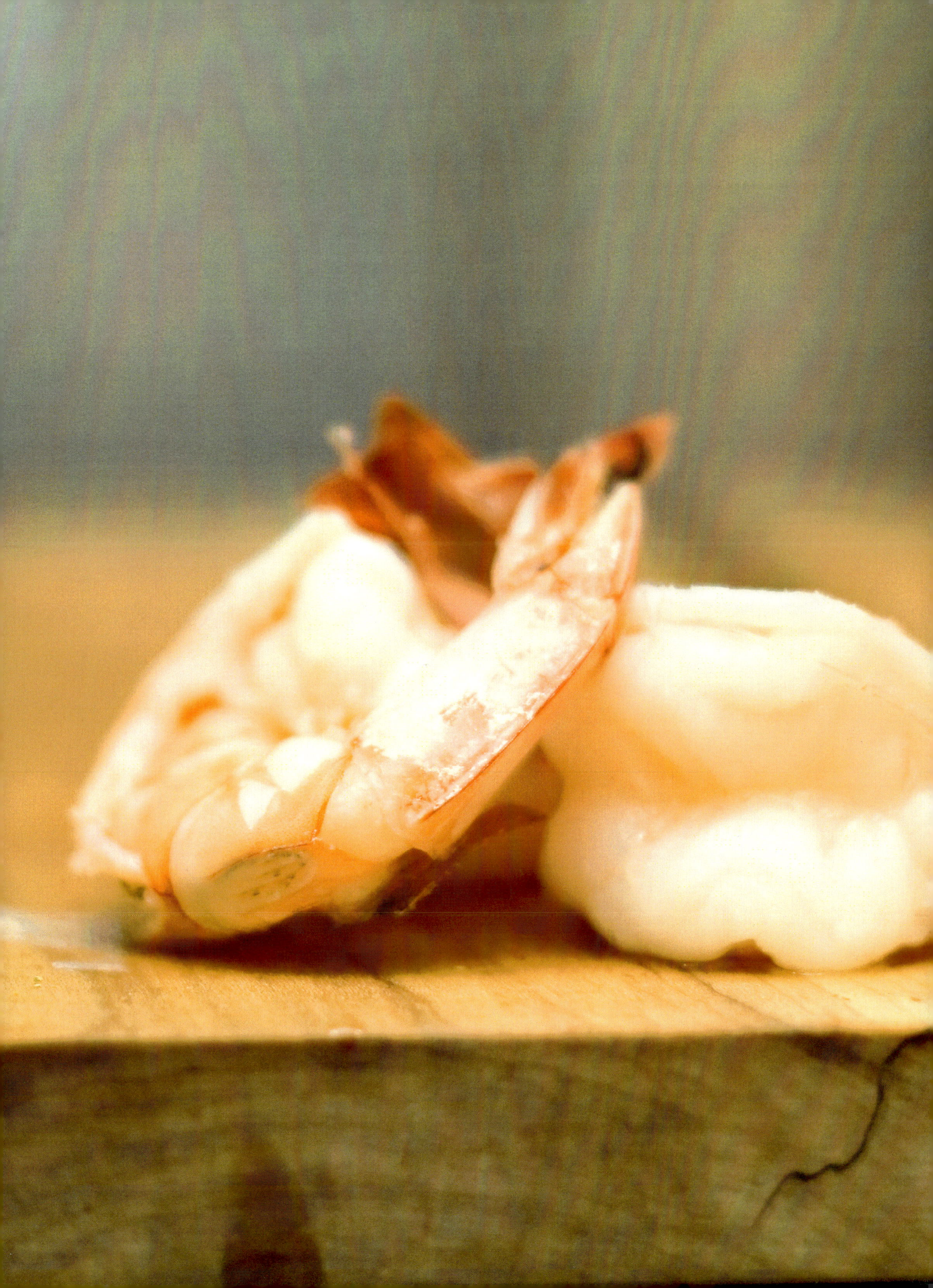

Stacked Salmon and Kale
(Calories: 340, 24 g protein, 10 g fat, 40 g carbohydrates)

Serves 4

1	Preheat broiler to 475° F	
2	Clean, peel and cut yam in quarters and steam for 20 minutes. Mash adding butter and half and half until smooth. Season with salt and pepper. Keep warm.	4 C. yam 2 T. butter 2 T. half and half (may use milk) ¼ t. sea salt ¼ t. pepper
3	Place fish on broiler pan and broil each side 4 minutes.	4 four oz. salmon fillets
4	Steam kale leaves for 4-8 minutes; drain and squeeze out excess water.	8 oz. kale, leaves only
5	On a dinner plate, place ¼ of the yam in center of plate. Layer with fish and kale and drizzle with balsamic vinegar. Serve.	1-2 T. balsamic vinegar

Greek Stuffed Steak

(Calories: 177, 21 g protein, 8 g fat, 20 g carbohydrate)

Serves 4-6

1	Steam the greens for 4 minutes drain. Combine in a bowl; set aside.	1 lb. kale or chard leaves only, chopped 1/3 C. shallot, chopped 1/3 C. pepperoncini peppers, chopped 2 T. breadcrumbs ½ t. sea salt 4 oz. goat cheese, crumbled
2	Trim the fat off the steak. Cut horizontally through center of steak, cutting to, but not through other side; open flat as you would a book. Place steak between two sheets of plastic; flatten to an even thickness, using a meat mallet or rolling pin.	1 (1½ lb.) flank steak (grass-fed if possible)
3	Spread spinach mixture over steak leaving a 1 inch margin around outside edges. Roll up jelly roll fashion and secure with heavy cooking string.	
4	Coat a large Dutch oven with oil and place over medium high heat. Brown steak well on all sides. Add tomato juice, broth, and oregano to pan; bring to a boil. Cover and reduce heat and simmer 1 ½ hours until tender, turning meat once. Add additional water if needed. Remove string and cut steak.	2 T. olive oil ½ C. tomato juice 1 (14 ½ oz.) can beef broth ½ t. oregano, dried ½ C. water (if needed) **Tip:** Serve with a green salad to complete the meal.

Bison (Buffalo) Cooking Tips
(Per/100g raw, trimmed: 22 g protein, 2 g fat)

Use lower temperatures for cooking as Bison is extra lean.

1 Steaks

Grill or BBQ 6 inches from heat source on medium high. Cook 4-6 minutes per side. Meat thermometer should read between 135° for rare to 145° for medium rare.

¾ to 1 inch thick *Steaks

2 Roast

In oven use uncovered pan with rack. Season as desired.

Cook at 275° (135°-145°F meat thermometer).

Preheat BBQ and turn off one side. Place roast on side that is turned off. Cook to rare 135°F or medium rare 145°F

Rib, Loin or Tenderloin

3 Pot Roast and Braising

Use pan with cover to create moist heat to cook. Brown in small amounts of oil. Simmer on top of stove until done. Fork should go into meat easily.

*Sirloin Tip, *Inside Round, Shoulder Brisket, Ribs
1-3 T. olive oil

*Marinate prior to cooking 8-24 hours

Tip: *Marinade: 1 ½ C. olive oil, ½ C. tarragon vinegar, ½ C. water, 1 8 oz. can tomato sauce, 1 t horseradish, 1 t. Worcestershire sauce, 1 t. sea salt, ½ t. pepper. Combine and pour over meat and refrigerate. (This marinade works great for beef as well.)

Chipotle-Marinated Pork Tenderloin
(Calories: 140, 24 g protein, 4 g fat, 2 g carbohydrates)

Serves 4

1	In a food processor or blender combine and set aside.	1 small can chipotle peppers in adobo sauce* 1 garlic clove, chopped 1/3 C. orange juice 3 T. lime juice 1 T. apple cider vinegar ¼ t. cumin 1 t. oregano, dried ¼ t. sea salt and pepper
2	Place pork tenderloins in plastic bag with sauce and marinate for at least 1 hour.	2 - 8 oz. pork tenderloins
3	Preheat grill to high heat. Remove the pork from the bag. Grill turning every 4-5 minutes for 15-20 minutes or until the instant-read thermometer reads 145° F.	
4	Transfer pork to cutting board and let sit before slicing.	
5	Can be refrigerated and sliced on greens with sliced fennel, grapefruit segments, sliced red onion and pumpkin seeds. Will keep refrigerated 2-3 days.	

Tip: * The chipotle peppers in adobo sauce is actually option green but it is less then 10% of the whole dish so I have left it in for flavor. This needs a side vegetable or the salad listed above with it for more carbohydrates.

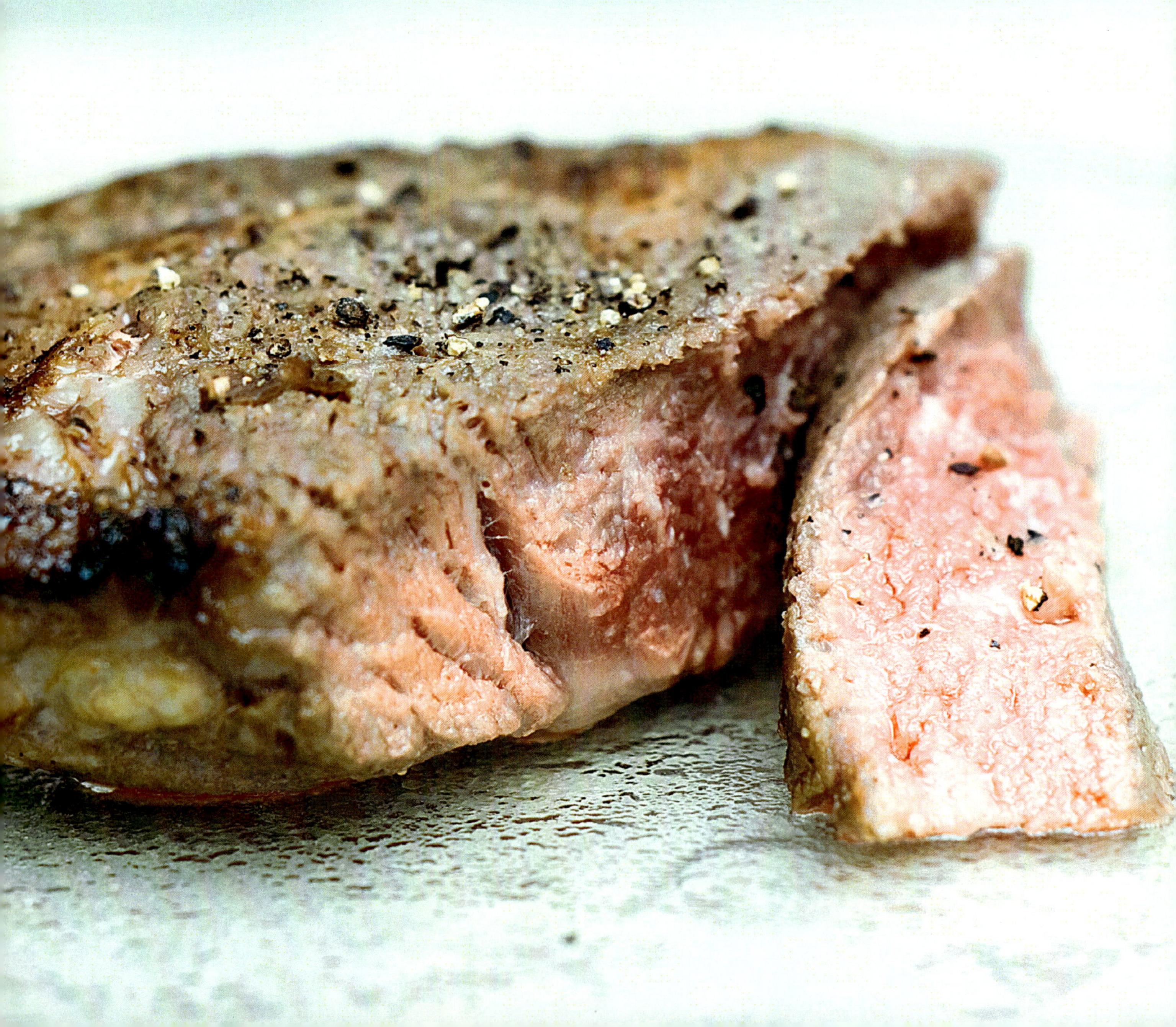

Nancy's Grass-Fed Beef Recipes

1 Baked Round Steak

Spread butter on Steak, sprinkle mushrooms over steak and salt and pepper. Wrap in 2 thicknesses of foil; place in covered roaster with rack. Bake in 325° oven for 2 hours.

Serves 6-8

¼ lb. raw butter
2 lb. round steak
4 oz. leeks, sliced
¼ t. sea salt
¼ t. pepper

2 Beef and Bacon Rollups

Combine all ingredients except the bacon. Make into 8 patties and surround each patty with a slice of bacon fastened with a toothpick. Broil or grill each side about 7 minutes. Serve on a Boston lettuce or a bun.

Serves 8

10 slices thin bacon
1 free-range egg, beaten
3 T. Worcestershire sauce
2 lb. ground beef
1 C. raw cheddar cheese, shredded
1 t. sea salt
½ t. pepper

3 Beef Kabobs

In a large bowl, whisk together oil and seasonings; add beef, and vegetables, tossing. Alternately thread beef with vegetables on 12 inch metal skewers. Broil or grill about 12-15 minutes turning often.

Serves 6-8

1 lb. grass-fed beef stew meat, cubed
1 medium zucchini, chopped in rounds
1 red bell pepper, cut in 1 ½ inch square
1 T. olive oil
2 t. Dijon-style mustard
1 t. honey
½ t. oregano, dried
¼ t. pepper

4 Chopped Steaks in Shallots Sauce

Finely chop half the shallots, thin slice remaining.

Combine chopped onion, ground beef and salt in large bowl and shape into four ½ inch patties. Heat oil in skillet and brown patties 10-12 minutes turning once. Remove from skillet; keep warm. Add sliced shallots and ¼ cup of beer to skillet; cook over medium heat 5 minutes, stirring occasionally. Combine gravy mix with remaining beer in a small bowl; mix until smooth and stir in thyme. Simmer until heated through and pour over patties. Serves 6-8

1¼ lb. ground beef patties
2-3 medium shallots, cut in half
¾ t. sea salt
¼ t. pepper
1 T. olive oil
1½ C. beer (12 ounces)
1 package (.87-.88 oz.)brown gravy mix
½ t. thyme, dried or 2 t. fresh chopped thyme

5   **Pot Roast with Vegetables**

Sprinkle roast with salt and pepper. Place shallots in the bottom of a 5-6 quart Crock Pot. Lay meat on top of the halved vegetables. Pour in the broth and Worcestershire sauce and whole herb; cover and cook on low for 5-6 hours. Remove the cover and add vegetables and salt and pepper cover and cook for an additional 1-1 ½ hours.

Serves 6-8

3-5 lb. top beef chuck roast, trimmed of excess fat

¼ t. sea salt

1-2 shallots quartered

zucchini, sliced in half

1-2 parsnips, sliced in half

1 C. beef broth

2 T. Worcestershire sauce

2 garlic cloves, whole

1 rosemary sprig or 1 t. dried

2 thyme sprigs or 1 t. dried

1 lb. new red potatoes

1 C. Brussels sprouts, cut in half

1 C. baby squash, cut in inch pieces

6   **Liver and Apples**

Sprinkle liver with salt and pepper. Melt butter in skillet. Cook liver about 3 minutes each side. Remove and keep warm. Add shallot and apple to skillet; cook until they are light brown. Serve over liver.

Serves 6-8

1 lb. sliced beef liver

½ t. salt

1/8 t. black pepper

¼ C. raw butter

1 large shallot, cut into thick slices

2 apples, cored , peeled and sliced

Pear and Cranberry Stuffed Pork Roast
(Calories: 170, 19 g protein, 7 g fat, 8 g carbohydrates)

Serves 4-6

1	Preheat oven to 400° F	
2	Heat oil in a large skillet over medium heat. Add onions, thyme, sage and garlic and sauté for 2 minutes until onion is tender. Stir in the broth scrapping the pan to loosen the brown bits. Cook until liquid is almost evaporated about 5 minutes.	1 T. olive oil ¼ C. onion diced ½ t. thyme, dried ½ t. sage. dried 2 cloves garlic, minced ½ C. chicken broth
3	Add the pear; cooking 5 minutes stirring often. Add cranberries and apple juice and cook 5 minutes. Remove from heat; let cool.	1 ½ C. pear, chopped ¼ C. dried cranberries ¼ C. apple juice
4	Unroll roast; sprinkle with salt and pepper. Spread pear mixture over roast leaving 2 inch margins around edges. Roll up jelly roll style securing with twine. Bake at 400° for 15 minutes	3 lb. pork tenderloin roast
5	Reduce temperature to 325° and cook for 1 hour or until the thermometer reads 160°.	
6	Let stand for 10 minutes before slicing.	

Tip: Serve with Green Beans and Mushrooms and a green salad.

Bacon-Wrapped Pork Tenderloin Filets
(Calories: 280, 22 g protein, 20 g fat, 5g carbohydrates)

Serves 4-6

1	Prepare pork: Trim off silver skin and fat and cut into 2" thick filets. Prepare the grill on medium high.	2 pork tenderloins (1 ½ lb. each)
2	To make the Chimichurri sauce; mince in food processor until smooth the first four ingredients and then add the oil, vinegar and water.	2 C. parsley leaves 2 T. garlic, chopped ½ t. pepper ½ t. red pepper flakes ½ C. olive oil ¼ C. white balsamic vinegar 2 T. water
3	Wrap bacon strips around each filet overlapping the ends and skewer each filet. Brush with Chimichurri sauce.	12 strips bacon, thin
4	Grill each side turning every 4 minutes basting with sauce each turn. Grill until internal temperature reaches 145° F, about 15 minutes. Serve with extra sauce.	

Tip: Serve with Black Bean and Corn Salad.

Enchiladas
(Calories: 350, 12 g protein, 10 g fat, 50 g carbohydrates)

1	Preheat oven to 375° F	May be frozen
2	Sauté chicken until done about 5 minutes each side. Cool and shred; set aside.	8-10 chicken breast, skinless boneless
3	Grate zucchini and add chopped shallots to the mixture; set aside.	2-4 zucchini 2-3 shallots, chopped
4	Grate the cheeses; set aside.	8 oz. mozzarella cheese
5	Place enchilada sauce in a pan and warm.	1 large can Enchilada sauce (Rosarita or similar)
6	Heat tortillas on the stove until warm.	12-18 corn tortillas
7	Dip the tortilla into the sauce and place in a large baking pan. Add chicken or meat, zucchini mixture and cheese in the center and roll up. Continue until all are filled.	
8	Pour remaining sauce over enchiladas; sprinkle any remaining cheese. Bake for 15-20 min.	

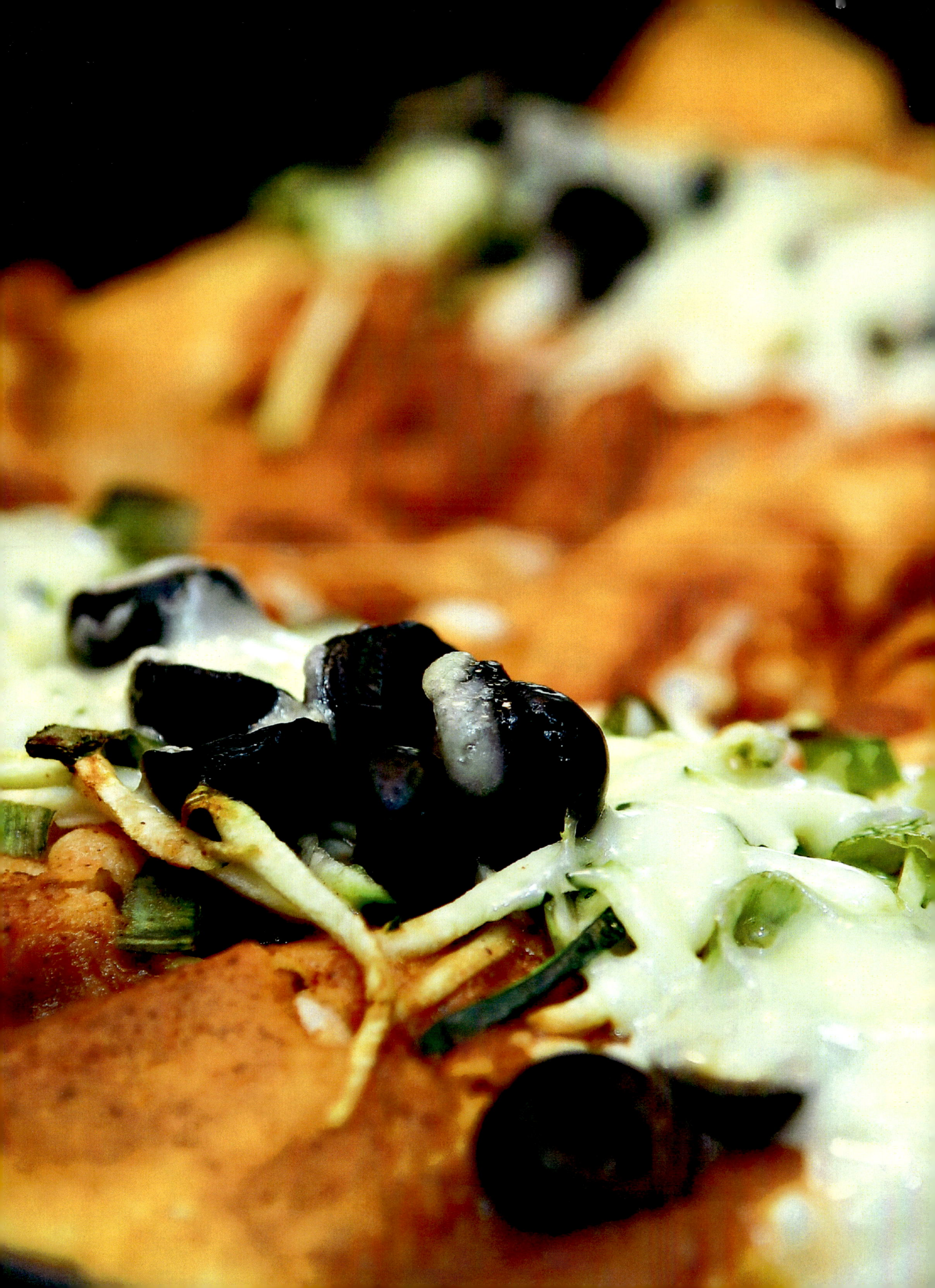

Raspberry-Rhubarb Pie Pg 106

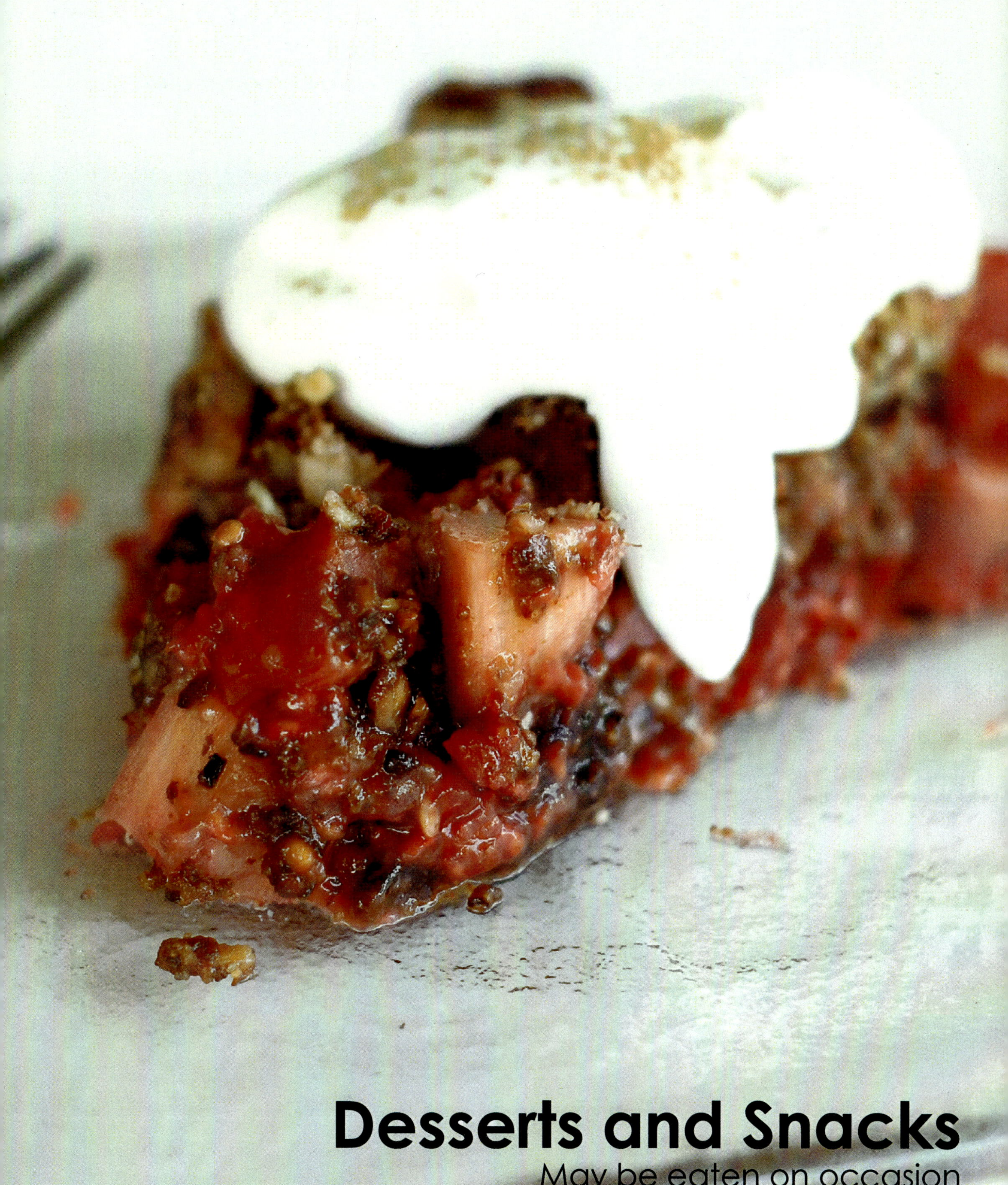

Desserts and Snacks
May be eaten on occasion

Pear Apple Crisp

(Calories: 200, 4 g protein, 4 g fat, 38 g carbohydrates)

Serves 12

1	Preheat oven to 400° F	
2	To make filling combine in a 2-quart baking dish all ingredients and set aside.	1 lb. organic apples. thinly sliced 1 lb. organic pears, thinly sliced 1 T. lemon juice ½ T. stevia (may use 2 T. maple syrup) 1 t. vanilla extract 1 T. arrowroot powder 1 t. cinnamon ½ C. organic unsweetened apple juice
3	To make the topping mix ingredients well and pour over filling.	½ C. rolled oats ½ C. almond meal ¼ C. coconut oil (liquefied) ¼ t. stevia or 1 T. maple syrup 1 C. toasted sunflower seeds, chopped
4	Cover dish with foil and bake for 45 minutes. Uncover and continue baking until golden brown about 20 minutes.	
5	May be eaten warm or at room temperature.	

Tip: This served with the yogurt dessert as a topping is delicious!

Peach Frozen Yogurt

(Serving 1/2 cup: 98 calories, 4 g protein, 2 g fat, 16 g carbohydrates)

Serves 4

1	Mix together in a bowl.	4 C. plain full fat yogurt 1 T. stevia or 2-3 T honey 1 t. vanilla extract
2	Mix the milk into the yogurt.	¾ C. whole organic milk
3	Thaw peaches slices and add to mixture using a blender or hand mixer, blend until smooth.	16 oz. of frozen peach slices
4	Pour into an ice cream maker and mix until thickened about 20-25 minutes.	
5	Spoon into cups and garnish with a mint leaf.	mint leaves

Raspberry-Rhubarb Pie
(Calories: 250, 47 g protein, 8 g fat, 40 g carbohydrates)

Serves 6-8

1	Preheat oven to 350° F	
2	Place tapioca in a coffee grinder or spice grinder; process until finely ground.	2 t. uncooked tapioca
3	Combine tapioca with ingredients in a bowl and let stand 10 minutes.	4½ C. fresh raspberries (about 24 ounces) ½ C. chopped fresh rhubarb (about 6 stalks) 1/3 C. maple syrup ¼ C. cornstarch ¼ C. apple juice 1/8 t. sea salt
4	To make the crust combine nuts, maple sprinkles and coconut oil in a food processor and process until paste is formed. Place in the bottom of a lightly oiled pie pan and gently press the dough into the pie dish. Bake 10 minutes.	½ C. sunflower seeds ½ C. almonds ½ C. oats 1 T. *maple sprinkles ½ C. almond meal ¼ C. coconut oil liquefied
5	Spoon raspberry mixture into crust and bake 40 minutes.	
6	While pie bakes, combine nuts, oatmeal, flour and sweetener in a food processor; pulse 10 times until mixture resembles coarse crumbs.	¼ C. almonds 1 T.*maple sprinkles ¼ C. oatmeal 5 T. coconut flour (may use wheat)
7	Increase oven temperature to 375° and sprinkle topping over pie. Bake 15 minutes more. Cool before serving.	

*Shady Maple Farms from www.citadelle-camp.coop.com

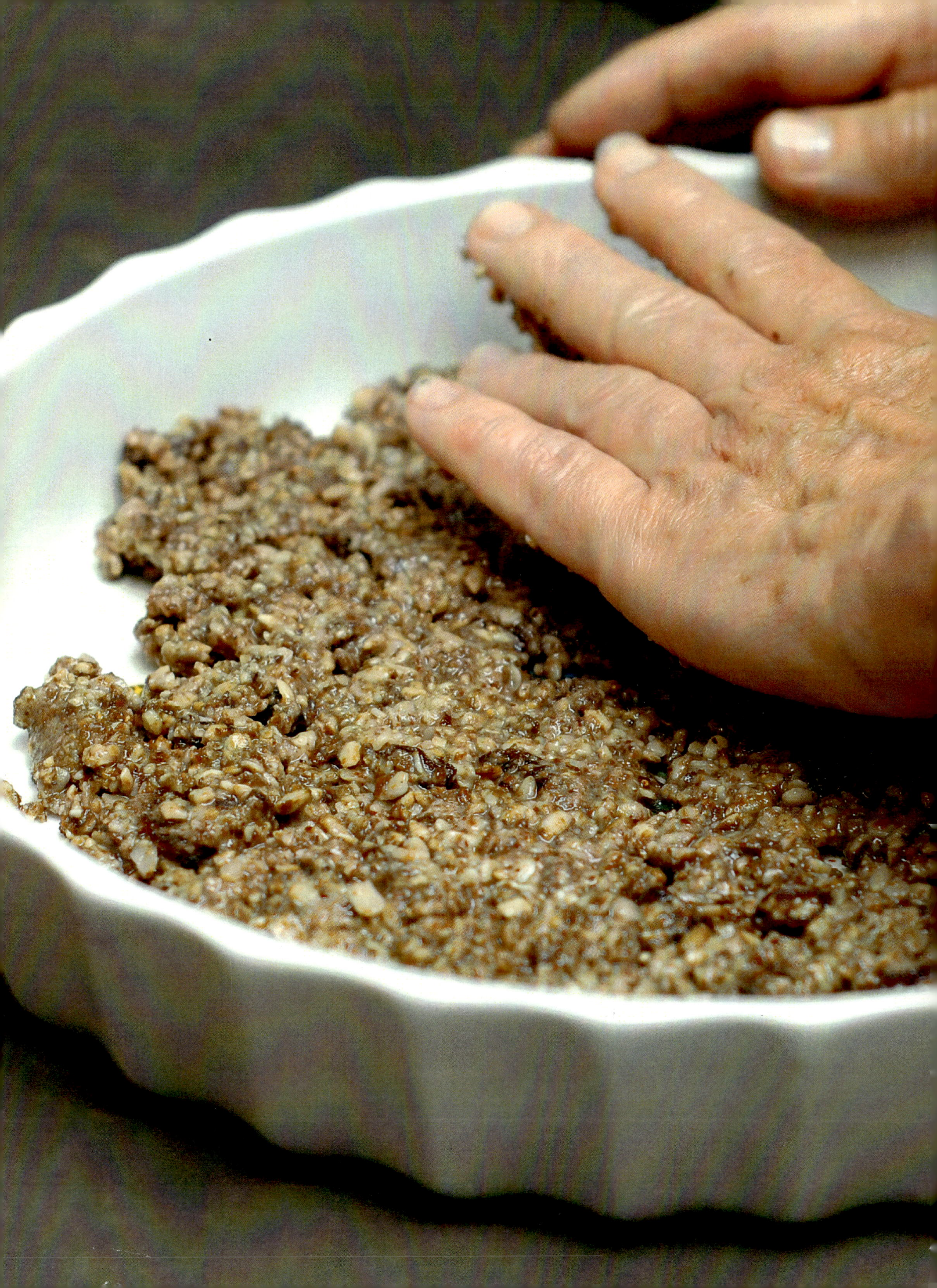

Energy Cookies
(Calories: 250, 4 g protein, 15 g fat, 24 g carbohydrates)

Makes 18-24 large cookies

1	Preheat oven to 350° F	
2	Mix dry ingredients. Set aside.	4 C. whole wheat pastry flour 1 C. pumpkin seeds 1 C. walnuts, chopped 1 C. macadamia nuts 2 C. semi-sweet chocolate chips 1 t. sea salt 4 t. baking powder
3	Mix wet ingredients.	1 C. currants soaked in 1 C. hot water 1 C. coconut oil, heated to liquid 1 C. maple syrup 2 T. vanilla extract 1-2 eggs (if needed)
4	Mix wet into dry ingredients. Batter should be stiff yet moist. Use egg slightly beaten if needed.	
5	Using a spoon form cookies and place on a cookie sheet. Flatten cookies slightly.	
6	Bake 15 minutes or until golden around the edges.	

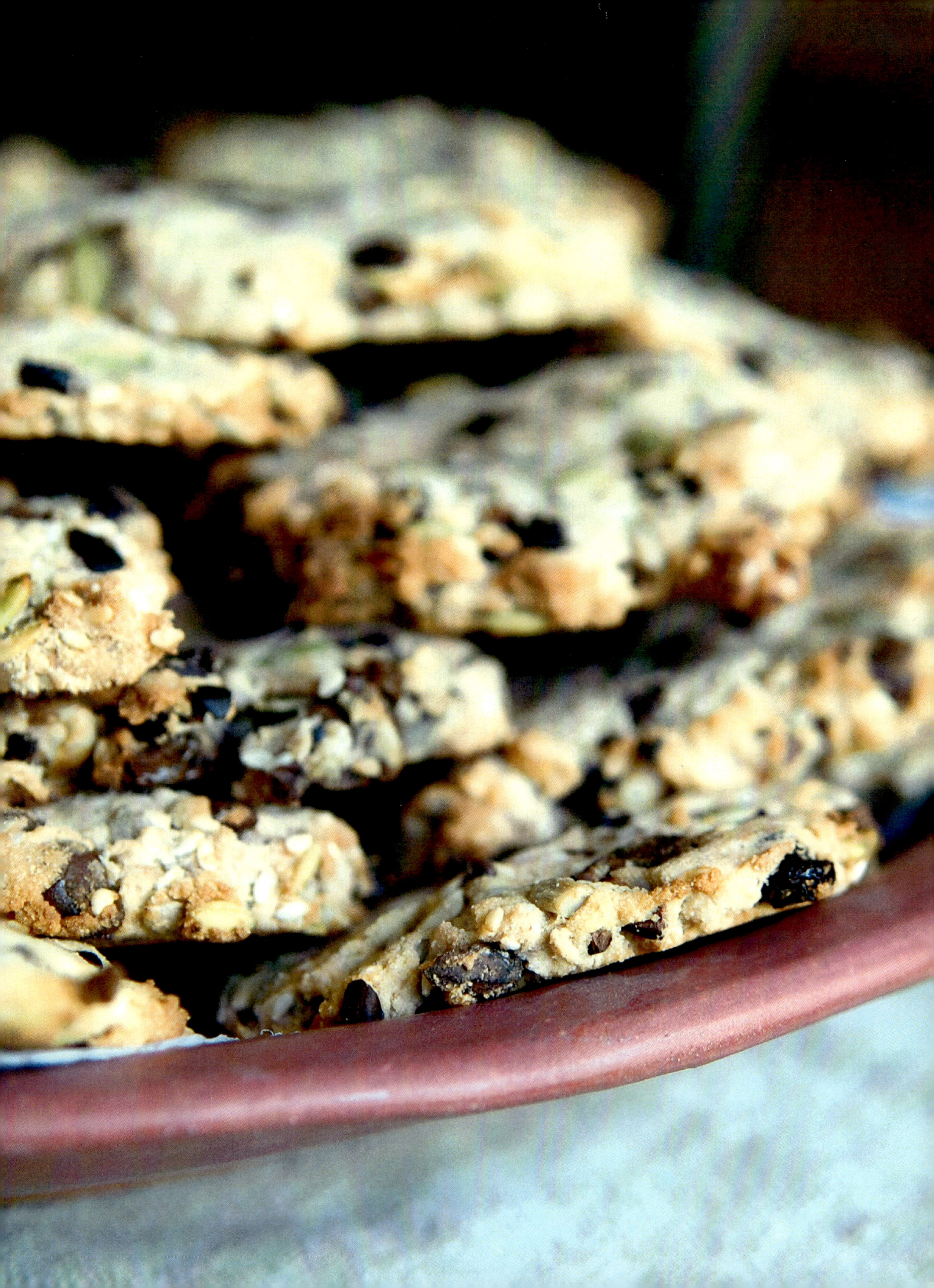

Apple Cashew Slice
(Calories: 120, 2 g protein, 5 g fat, 17 g carbohydrates)

Serves 6-8

1	Preheat oven to 375° F	
2	Blend in food processor or blender.	¼ C. coconut oil, warmed to liquid 2 medium green apples, grated ½ t vanilla extract 1 t. cinnamon ¼ t. cardamom
3	Add to mixture and blend.	½ C. cashews
4	Add to mixture and blend.	1 C. dry unsweetened coconut flakes ½ C. rolled oats 1 pear, grated
5	Pour into a greased 9 inch baking pan. Bake for 25-30 minutes.	
6	Cool; cut into wedges.	

Tip: Top with plain yogurt or whipped cream (sweetened with stevia and vanilla extract) and sprinkle toasted unsweetened coconut flakes.

Energy Trail Mix for #3-A
(1/4 cup serving: Calories 200, 9 g protein, 18 g fat, 18 g carbohydrates)

Serves 26

1	In a medium size bowl mix all the ingredients.

½ C. dried wild blueberries
1 C. *coca nibs
1 C. almonds, whole, raw
1 C. cashews, whole, raw
1 C. hulled raw sunflower seeds
1 C. pistachios
1 C. pine nuts

May add:
½ t. stevia or maple sprinkles
¼ t. sea salt

*cocoa nibs can be used in recipes or for a snack when chocolate taste buds need satisfying. May be found at your health food store.

2	Store in a covered jar and keep in a dark place or refrigerate.

1. Yogurt Dessert or
2. Ricotta Cheese Dessert

Serves 4-6

1 Yogurt Dessert

In bowl mix yogurt with stevia and vanilla extract until smooth.

In 4-6 custard cups place ½ cup chopped berries top with ½ cup yogurt mixture and sprinkle with ½ T toasted nuts, serve.

15 oz. Greek plain yogurt , full fat
1 T. stevia powder or 2-3 T honey
1 t. vanilla extract
1 lb. fresh berries
¼ C. chopped nuts, toasted

2 Ricotta Cheese Dessert

Mix ricotta in bowl with stevia or honey and vanilla.

Grate the chocolate and gentle fold into cheese mixture.

Place ½ cup in small cup or glass and top with a macaroon cookie.

1 pt. ricotta cheese
1 T. stevia or 2-3 T honey
1 t. vanilla extract
1 squares 72% dark chocolate
4-6 macaroon cookies

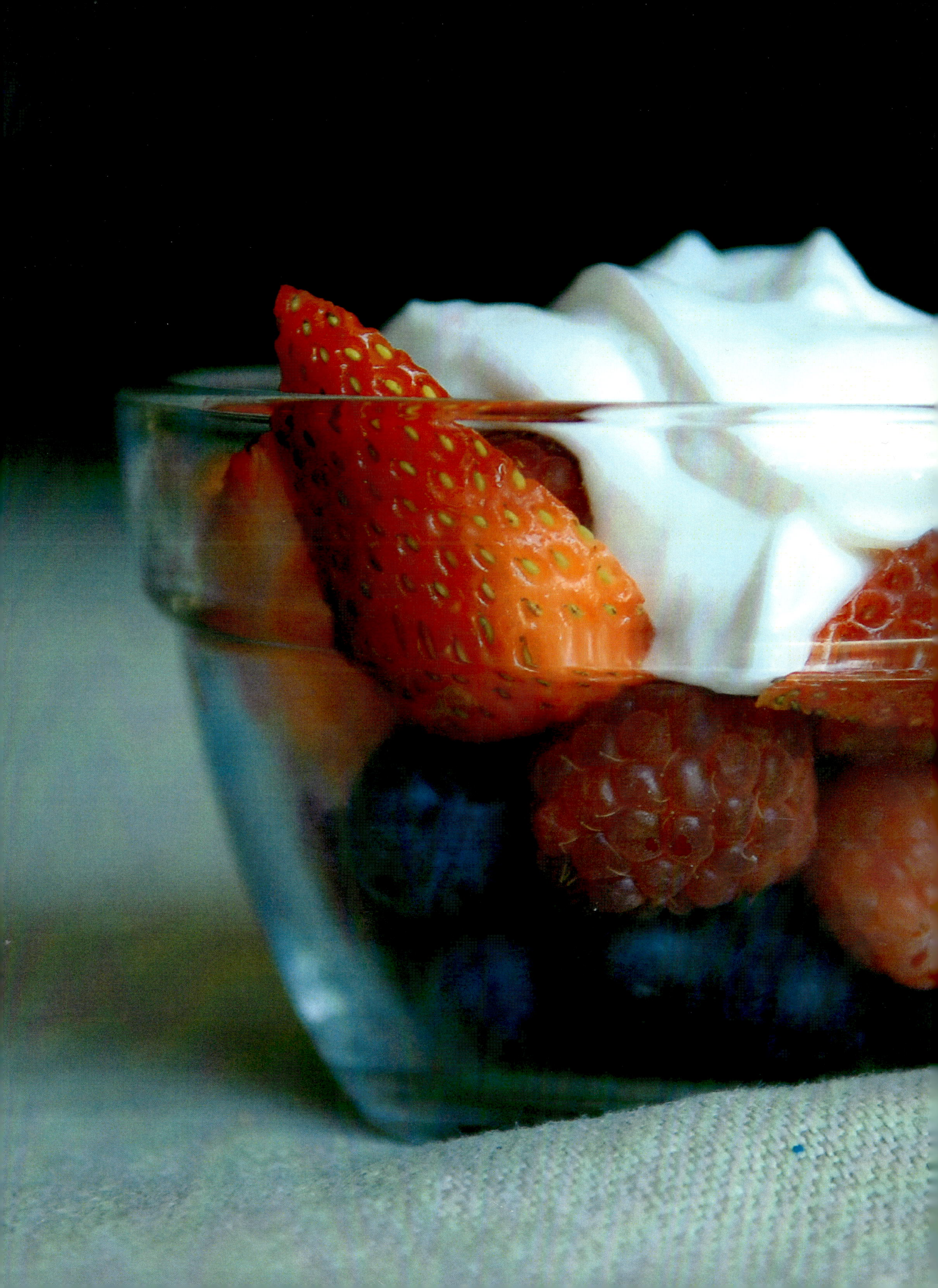

Glossary

Arrowroot: A white powder used for thickening sauces. It becomes clear when cooked.

Arugula (Rocket Rugula): An elongated green leaf with a peppery sharp almost mustardy flavor. It can be used in place of spinach in soups and vegetables stews.

Barley: An ancient grain that is very digestible. Hulled barley is superior over pearl barley but it requires longer cooking time and is chewier.

Bragg Liquid Aminos: This is a very tasty soy sauce-like condiment made by extracting amino acids from organic soybeans. It is not fermented, making it an ideal seasoning for those who suffer from yeast sensitivities. You can find it in most health food stores.

Capers: Pickled flower buds. Adds a salty taste; always rinse before using.

Coconut oil: It is a saturated fat that cooks at high temperatures without smoking.

Couscous: A staple of North Africa is made of durum wheat stripped of the bran and germ. Try and get whole wheat couscous which has the bran. It is very quick to cook in less than five minutes.

Curry Paste: A concentrated seasoned mixture of red chilies and spices found in oriental and eastern foods. It can be very hot.

Curry Powder: A blend of spices with degrees of "heat" from maker to maker. Most curry powders have the following: cumin, coriander, mustard seeds, fenugreek, red chilies, black pepper, and turmeric.

Cardamom: A spice found in curry powders. It adds a sweet-spiciness to baked goods and cuts through the flavor and texture of oil.

Fennel: Has a sweet licorice taste. The plant looks like celery. Sliced in salads or soups it adds a delicate taste. I prefer the fennel raw or I like to add at the end of the dish to retain the flavor.

Fish Sauce: Made from salted anchovies. May use in place of salt or soy sauce. It has a very pungent aroma, but the aroma will mellow with cooking.

Flax Seeds: Have a high omega-3 fatty acid ratio and make for a good binder in baked goods. They have a sweet nutty flavor. Because of their high oil content, the seeds tend to go rancid. Store them whole in the freezer for up to three months and grind as needed. They have a laxative effect so eat flax in moderation.

Garam Masala: A blend of dry roasted spices used in Indian cooking. Combination of about twelve spices including: black pepper, cinnamon, cloves, coriander, cumin, fennel, mace and nutmeg. Add towards the end of cooking for more flavors.

Ghee: Clarified butter used in Indian and Middle Eastern cooking. It can be made by melting unsalted butter and removing the scum and foam from the top as it melts.

Ginger, fresh: Buy ginger fresh with smooth skin and store in your refrigerator in a brown bag sealed tightly. To use the root cut a piece and grate or slice. It is not necessary to peel the root unless it is dark brown and shriveled. It should have plenty of juice which can be added to the dish as well. If the recipe calls for fresh ginger you can not substitute dried as it has an entirely different flavor.

Goatein protein powder: A protein powder made from pre-digested goats milk. Made by Garden of Life.

Gomasio: Ground sesame seeds and sea salt.

Great Northern Beans: These are white beans harvested in the Mid-west.

Hemp protein powder: Contains all essential amino acids along with a balance of omega 6 and omega 3 in a ratio of 3 to 1. It also contains GLA for hormone balancing.

Lentils: A very ancient legume. There are many varieties. Brown have a peppery taste, green have a milder taste and my favorite are the French variety that are smaller, sweeter and hold its shape in soups and salads.

Quinoa: Native grain from the Andes and about the size of a sesame seed. Has higher protein and amino acid profile. Be sure and rinse well to remove the bitter saponin coating (believed to be a natural insect repellant) before cooking and drain it thoroughly.

Rhubarb: Considered a fruit it is really a vegetable with red stalks and poisonous leaves. Select medium–thick stalks to slender so they are less stringy; can be stored in the refrigerator for one week sealed in a plastic bag. For cooking rinse well and cut off the ends and slice as directed.

Sea salt: Evaporated seawater which leaves trace minerals lost in refined salt. Has less sodium.

Soba Noodles: Buckwheat noodles. Generally, have other ingredients. I prefer the Eden Foods' brand. The Japanese technique of adding ½ cup of cold water to the boiling water twice during cooking time allows the middle of the noodle to cook thoroughly before the outside becomes soft and mushy.

Spelt: An ancient grain with a texture very similar to wheat. Some people who have sensitivity to wheat may be able to tolerate spelt.

Stevia: Natural sweetener from a plant grown in South America. It is ten times sweeter than sugar so use less.

Tamari: Type of naturally fermented soy sauce that takes a year to ferment. I prefer the organic wheat free type.

Tahini: Sesame butter; a rich peanut-buttery paste used in Middle Eastern and Asian cooking.

Tobasco Sauce: A well known brand name of a hot sauce used in vegetable or meat dishes.

Whey protein powder: Lactose free protein made from cow dairy. Use only good quality without any other ingredients or additives.

Legends, Weights and Measures

pinch = less then ¼ teaspoon
t.= teaspoon
T.= Tablespoon
C. = Cup
oz. = ounce
pt. = pint
lb. = pound
qt. = quart

To convert to metric

1 Cup = 250 ml
1 Tablespoon = 15 ml (Australia it would be 20 ml)
1 teaspoon = 5 ml

Oven setting equivalents

	Fahrenheit	Celsius	Gas regulo No
Very cool	225-275°	110-140	¼-1
Cool	300-325°	150-160	2-3
Moderate	350-375°	180-190	4-5
Hot	400-450°	200-260	6-8
Very Hot	475-500°	250-260	9-10

Grams to Ounces: These are converted to the nearest round number.

25=1	50=2	75=3	100=3.5	125=4	150=5
175=6	200=7	225=8	250=9	275=10	300=10.5
325=11	350=12	400=14	425=15	450=16	

1 kilogram= 1000 grams= 2lb. 4 oz.

Index

Apples
        Pear Apple Crisp, 104
        Apple Coconut Flour Nut Muffins, 29
        Apple Cashew Slice, 110
Bacon
        Bacon-wrapped Pork Tenderloin Filets, 99
Banana
        Protein Smoothies, 24
Beans, Black
        Black Bean and Corn Salad, 42
        Black Bean Chili, 60
Beans, Northern white
        Chicken and Spinach Soup with Fresh Pesto, 54
Beef
        Nancy's Grass-Fed Beef Recipes, 95
        Greek Stuffed Steak, 91
        Black Bean Chili, 60
Bison, 92
Blueberry
        Protein Smoothies, 24
        Yogurt Dessert, 112
Broccoli
        Rolled Chicken Stuffed with Vegetables, 85
Chicken
        Chicken Bone Broth, 49
        Chicken and Spinach Soup, 54
        Chicken Crusted in Almond, 82
        Chicken Curry, 80
        Chicken with Capers, 81
        Orange-ginger Chicken, 84
        Enchiladas, 100
        Rolled Chicken Stuffed with Vegetables, 85
        Rolled Chicken Stuffed with Vegetables, 86
        South of the Border Soup, 52
        Tom Ka Kai Soup, 51
Desserts
        Apple Cashew Slice, 110
        Energy Cookies, 108
        Energy Trail Mix, 111
        Peach Frozen Dessert, 105
        Pear Apple Crisp, 104
        Raspberry-Rhubarb Pie, 106
        Ricotta Cheese Dessert, 112
        Yogurt Dessert, 112
Eggs
        Asparagus Mushrooms over Eggs, 23
        Mini Mushroom and Sausage Quiches, 26
        Salmon Omelet, 28
        Sausage Mushroom Frittata, 27
Fish
        Salmon Omelet, 28
        Stacked Salmon and Kale, 90
        Salmon Cakes, 87
        Shrimp Jambalaya, 88

Muffins
  Apple Coconut Flour Muffins, 29
  Zucchini Muffins, 30
Mushrooms
  Mini Mushroom and Sausage Quiches, 26
  Asparagus and Mushrooms over Eggs, 23
  Tom Ka Kai Soup, 51
  Green Beans with Mushrooms, 71
  Cheese and Spinach Stuffed Portobello, 66
Nuts and Seeds
  Energy Trail Mix, 111
Pancakes
  Almond Pancakes, 22
Pears
  Pear and Cranberry Stuffed Pork Roast, 98
  Pear Apple Crisp, 104
Pork
  Mini Mushroom and Sausage Quiches, 26
  Prosciutto wrapped Broccoli, 67
  Bacon-wrapped Pork Tenderloin Filets, 99
  Pear and Cranberry Stuffed Pork Roast, 98
  Chipotle-Marinated Pork Tenderloin, 93
Potato
  Twice Baked Potatoes, 77
Raspberry
  Protein Smoothie, 24
  Raspberry-Rhubarb Pie, 106
Salads
  Artichoke and Ripe Olive with Tuna Salad, 44
  Black Bean and Corn Salad, 42
  Cold Asparagus with Sesame-ginger Vinaigrette, 36
  Fresh Fig Salad with Toasted Walnuts, 34
  Lentil Salad, 40
  Papaya and Walnut Green Salad, 35
  Quinoa Corn Salad, 41
  Santa Barbara Salad, 38
  Tuna Dip, 37
Salmon
  Salmon Omelet, 28
  Salmon Cakes, 87
Shrimp
  Shrimp Jambalaya, 88
Smoothies
  Basic Berry, 24
  Creamy Monkey, 24
  Reese's Pieces, 24
  Tropical Delight, 24
  Raspberry Delight, 24
Sausage
  Mini Mushroom and Sausage Quiches, 26
Soups
  Cauliflower Brie Soup, 59
  Coconut Curry, 56
  Chicken Bone Broth, 49
  Chicken and Spinach, 54

Lentil Vegetable, 50
Mushroom Barley and Beef Soup, 53
Split Pea and Ham, 57
Split Pea with Spicy Yogurt, 58
Tom Ka Kai , 51
Vegetable Broth #2, 48
South of the Border, 52

Turkey

Mini Mushroom and sausage Quiches, 26
Black Bean Chili, 60
Stuffed Butternut Squash, 73

Vegetables

Blue Cheese-Walnut Broccoli, 72
Brussels sprouts with Bacon-Balsamic Vinaigrette, 70
Cheese and Spinach Stuffed Portobello, 66
Green Bean with Mushrooms, 71
Green Beans with Pecans, 68
Green Bean Pate with Basil, 68
Mashed Cauliflower "Potatoes", 76
Mediterranean Vegetable Quinoa, 75
Mushroom Spinach Stuffed Summer Squash, 74
Prosciutto Wrapped Broccoli, 67
Restaurant Green Beans, 68
Sautéed Vegetables, 64
Stuffed Butternut Squash, 73
Twice Baked Potato, 77

Resources

US Wellness Meats
Grass fed beef, lamb, bison and free range poultry online store:
(877) 383-0051
www.uswellnessmeats.com

Great Alaska Seafood
Wild caught seafood delivered to your door. (866) 262-8846
www.great-alaskan-seafood.com

Tropical Traditions
Organic coconut oil and flour and other items.
Mail order to: P.O.Box 333, Springville, CA. 93265
www.tropicaltraditions.com

Lydia's Organics
Vegan-Gluten Free-Raw snacks. Phone: 415-258-9678 Fax: 415-258-9623
Convenient alternatives to commercial snacks, crackers, cereals and bars.
www.lydiaorganics.com

Julian Bakery
Organic wheat-free, preservative free breads. Phone 1-800-98-BREAD
www.julianbakery.com

Ultra-Life/Synergistics
Supplements , Celtic Salt, household and miscellaneous
Phone: 800-323-3842 Fax: 618-594-7712
www.ultralifeinc.com

Nantucket Rubs and Spices
Rubs and spices
www.nantucketoffshore.com

La Nogalera Walnut Oil
Walnut oil
www.langalerawalnutoil.com

Shady Maple Farms
Maple syrup products and farm co-op
www.citadelle-camp.coop.com

Coconut Secret
Organic coconut products including Coconut Nectar, Coconut Crystals,
Coconut Aminos, Coconut Vinegar and other products. 1-888-369-3393
www.coconutsecret.com